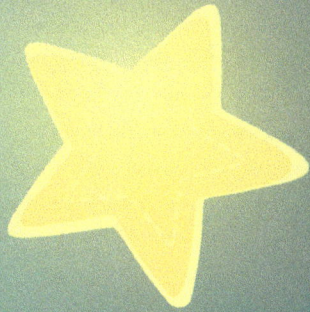

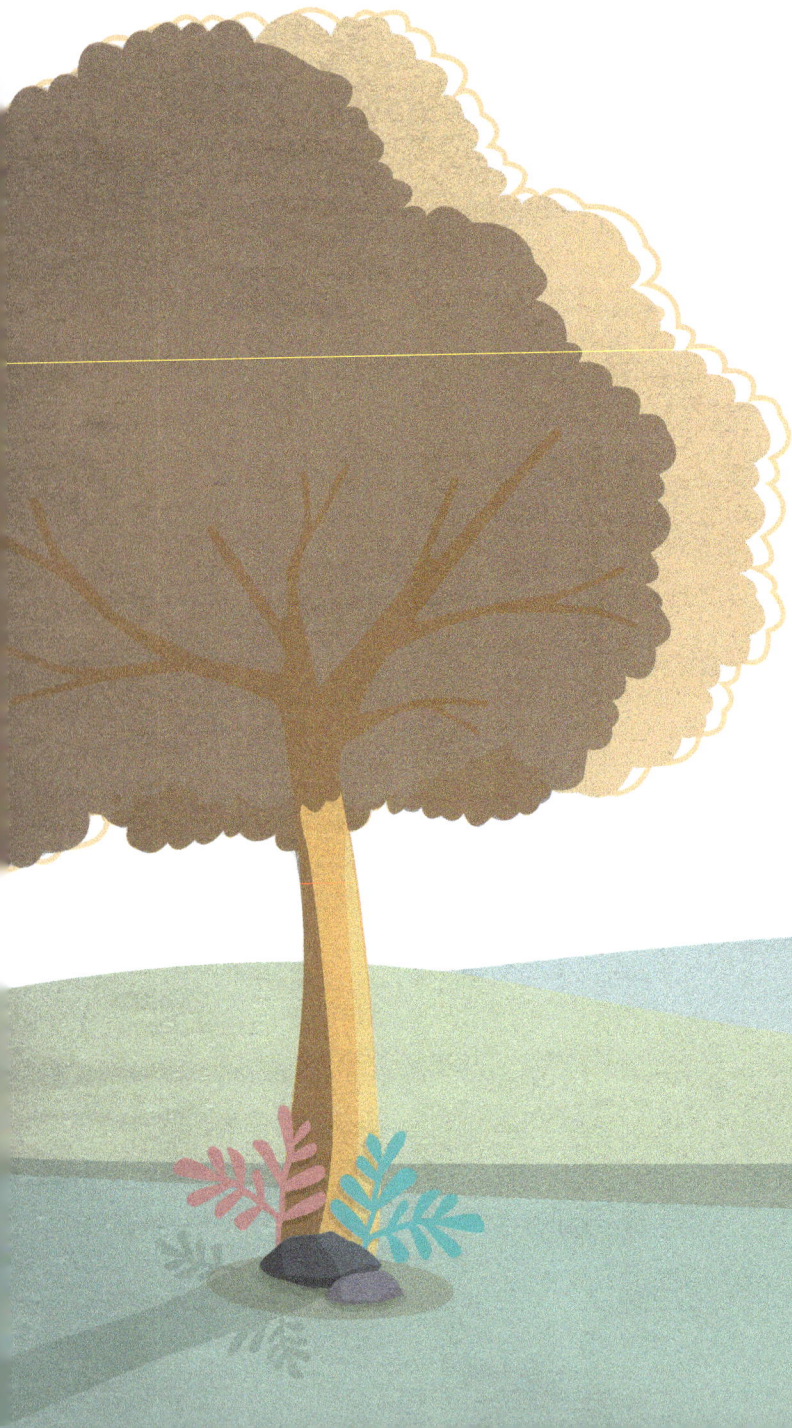

Cristina Cortés

HOW CAN I GET OUT OF HERE?

Zuzene Seminario
Daiana Etxeberria

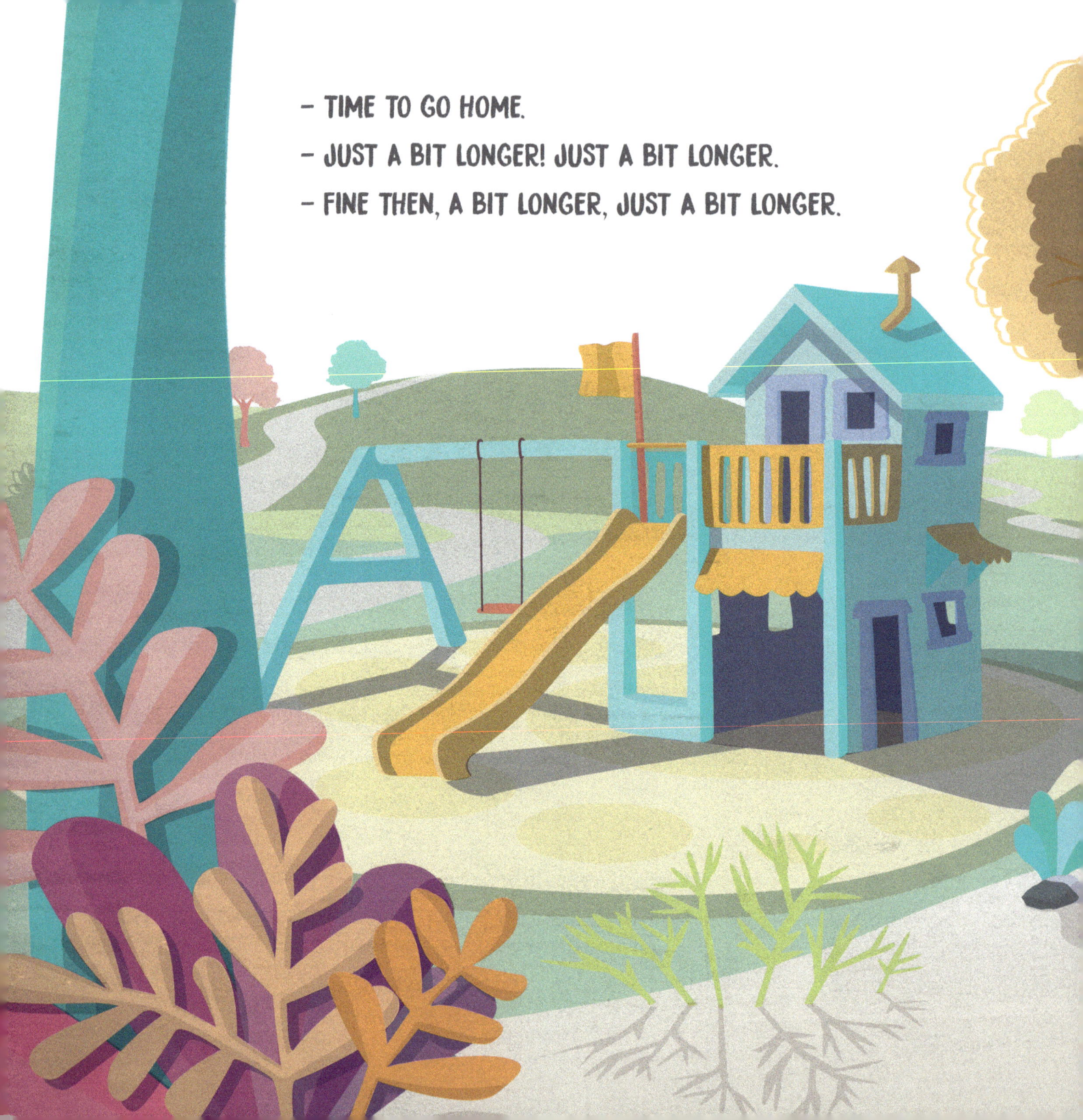

– TIME TO GO HOME.

– JUST A BIT LONGER! JUST A BIT LONGER.

– FINE THEN, A BIT LONGER, JUST A BIT LONGER.

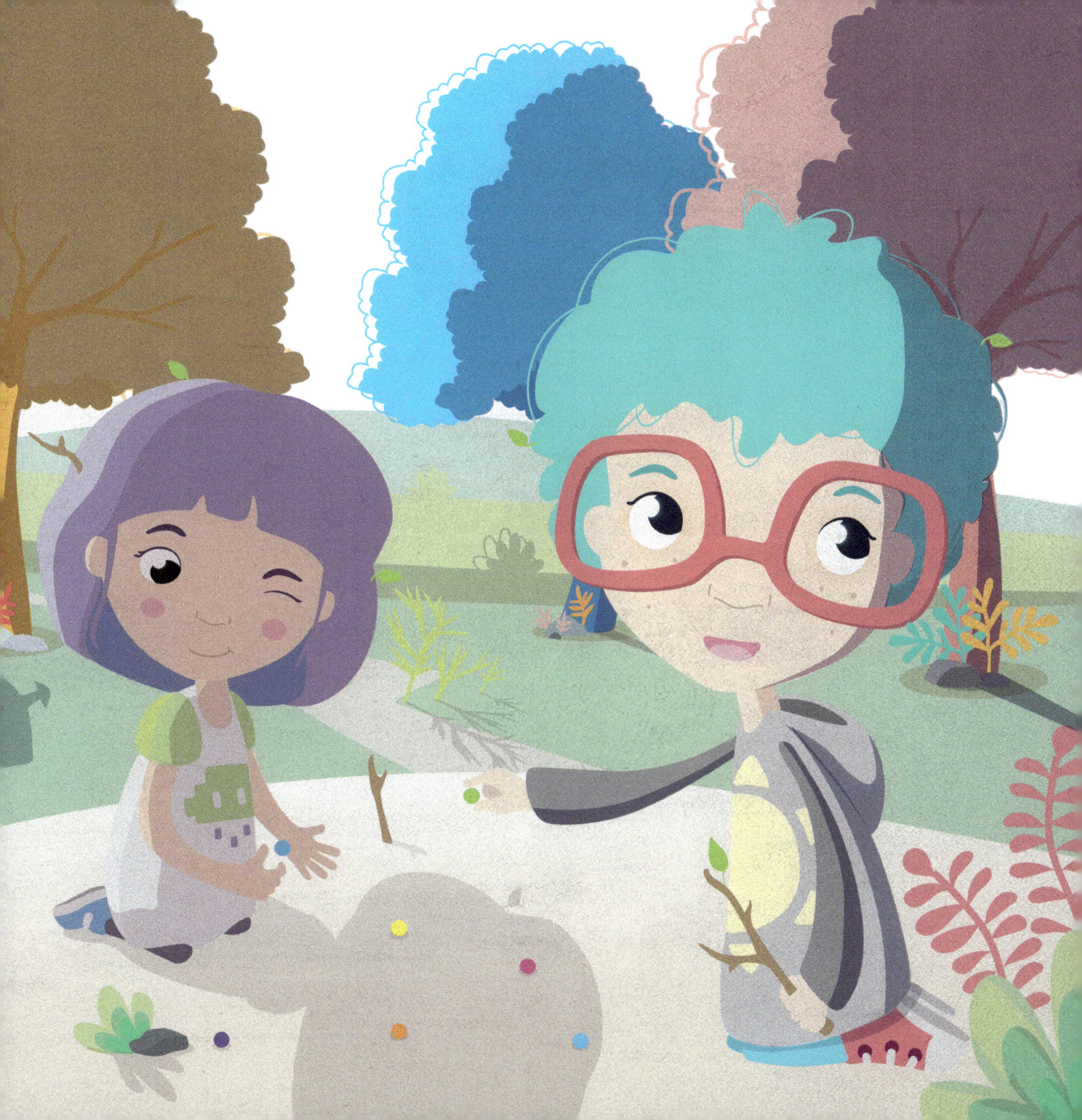

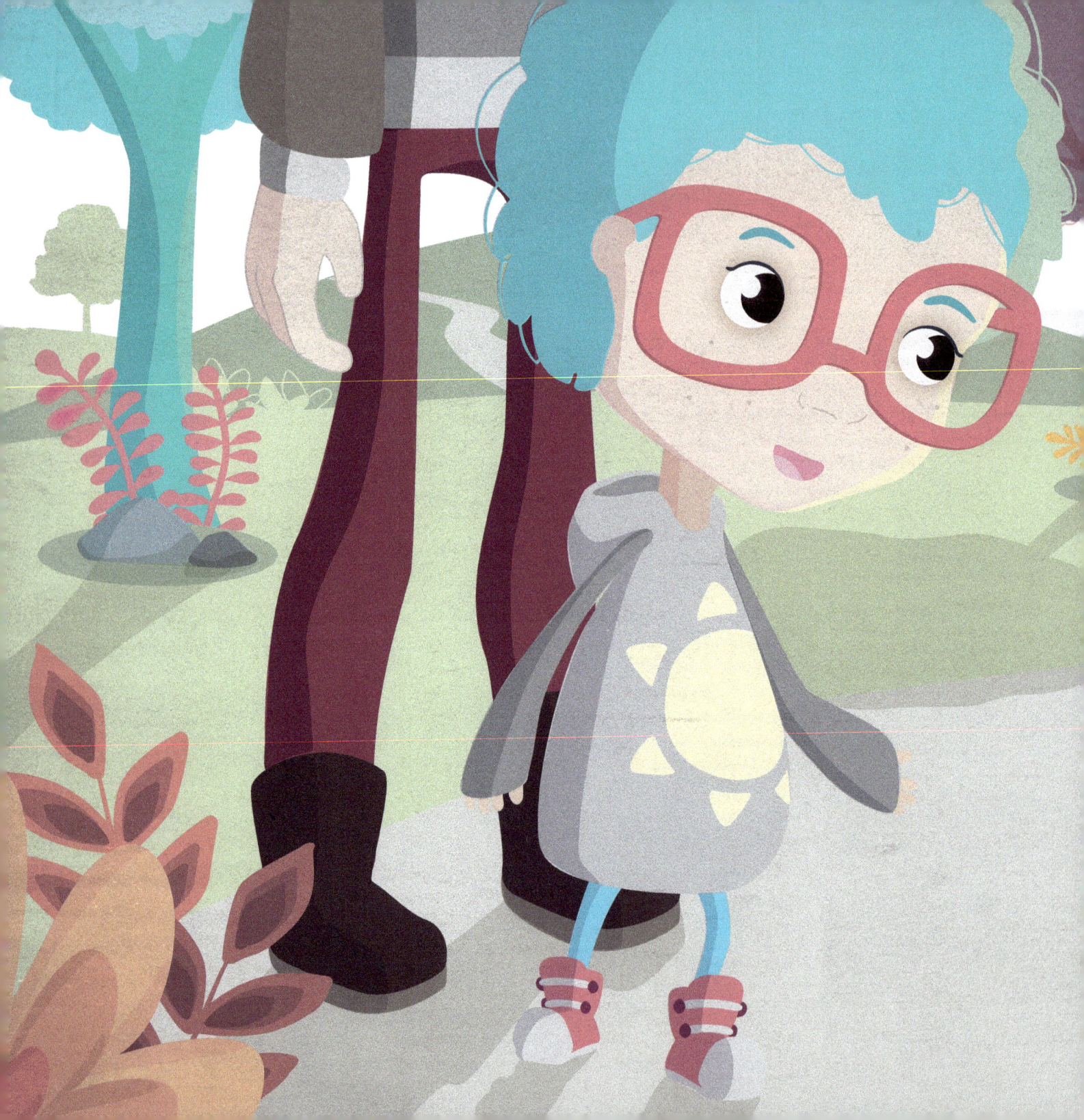

– I WANT A DOG, A LITTLE DOGGY.
  A BIT MORE. A BIT MORE. A BIT MORE.
– JUST A BIT MORE.

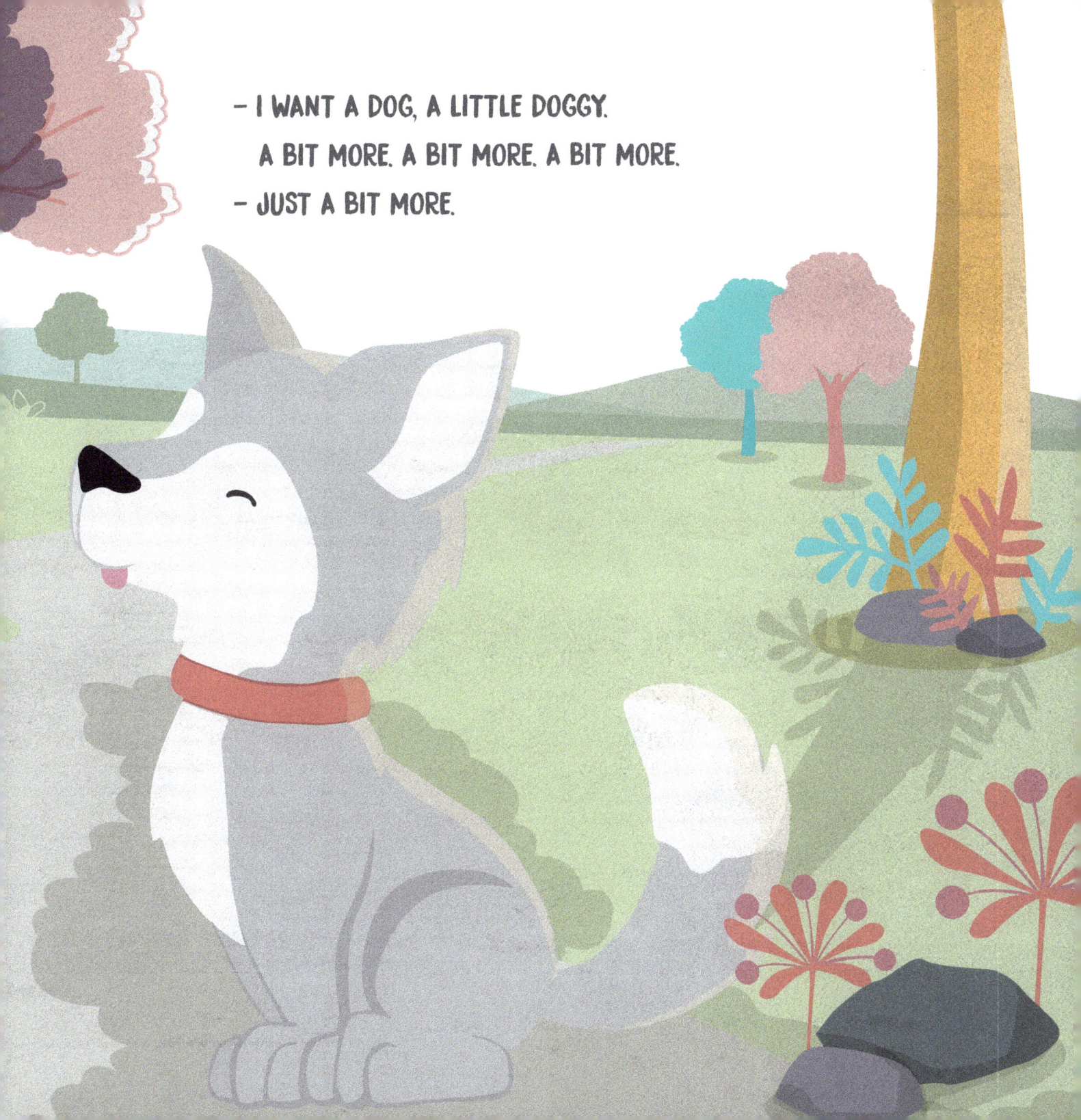

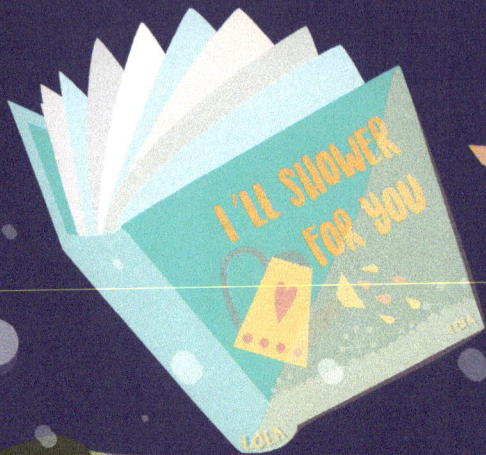

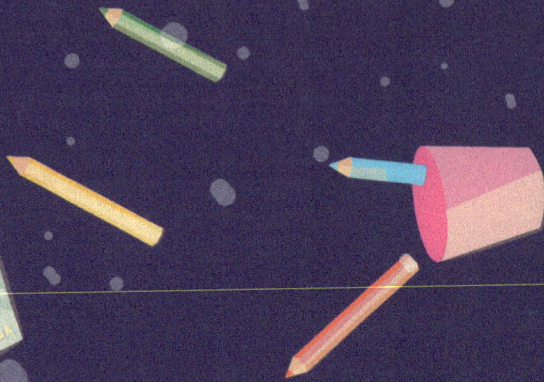

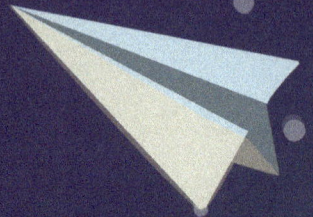

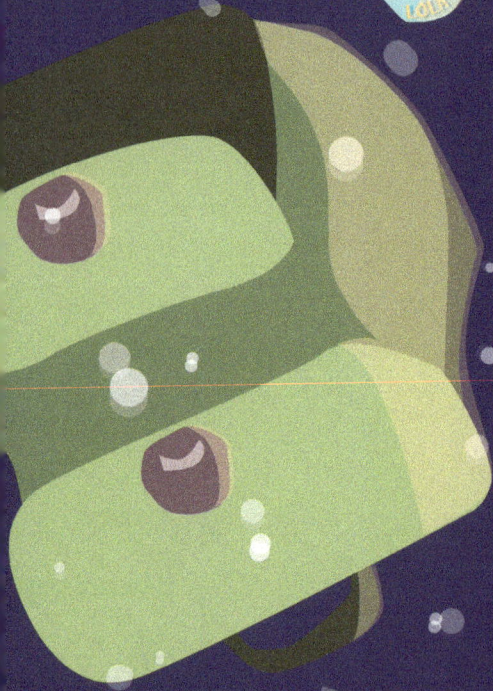

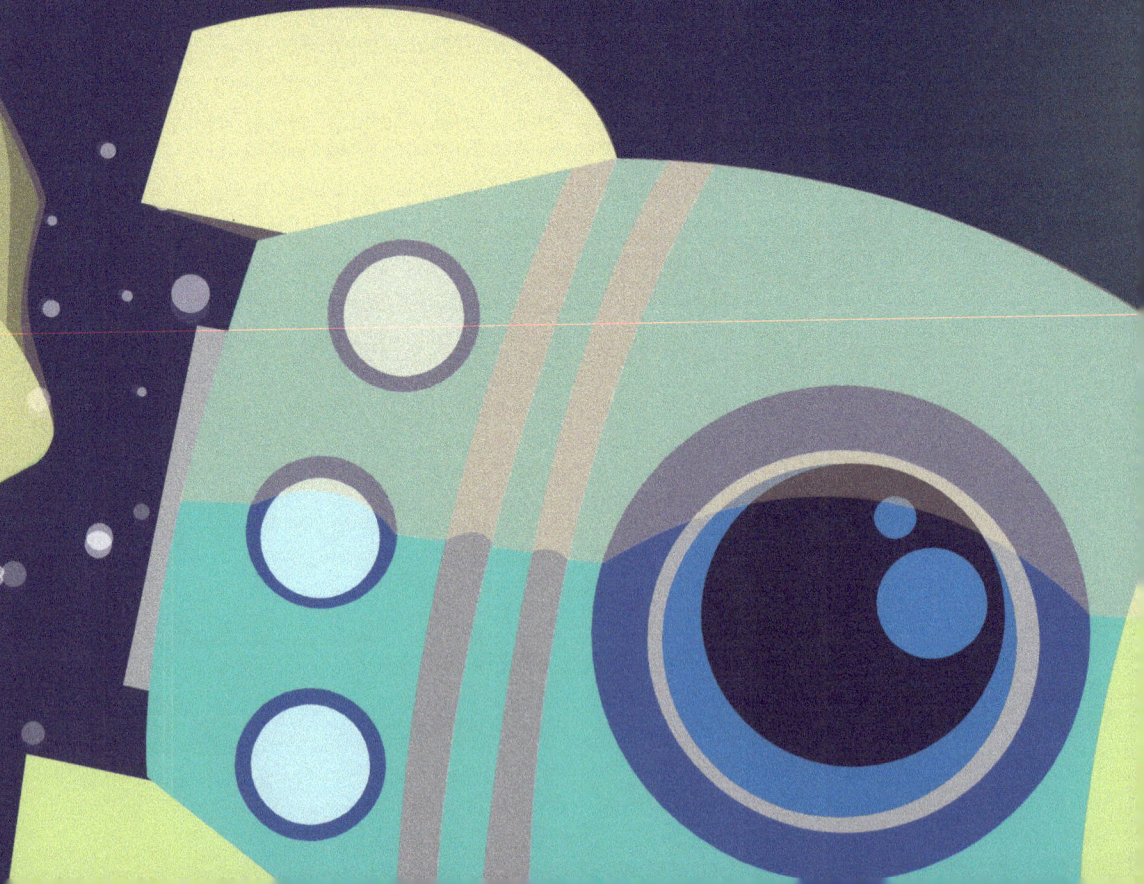

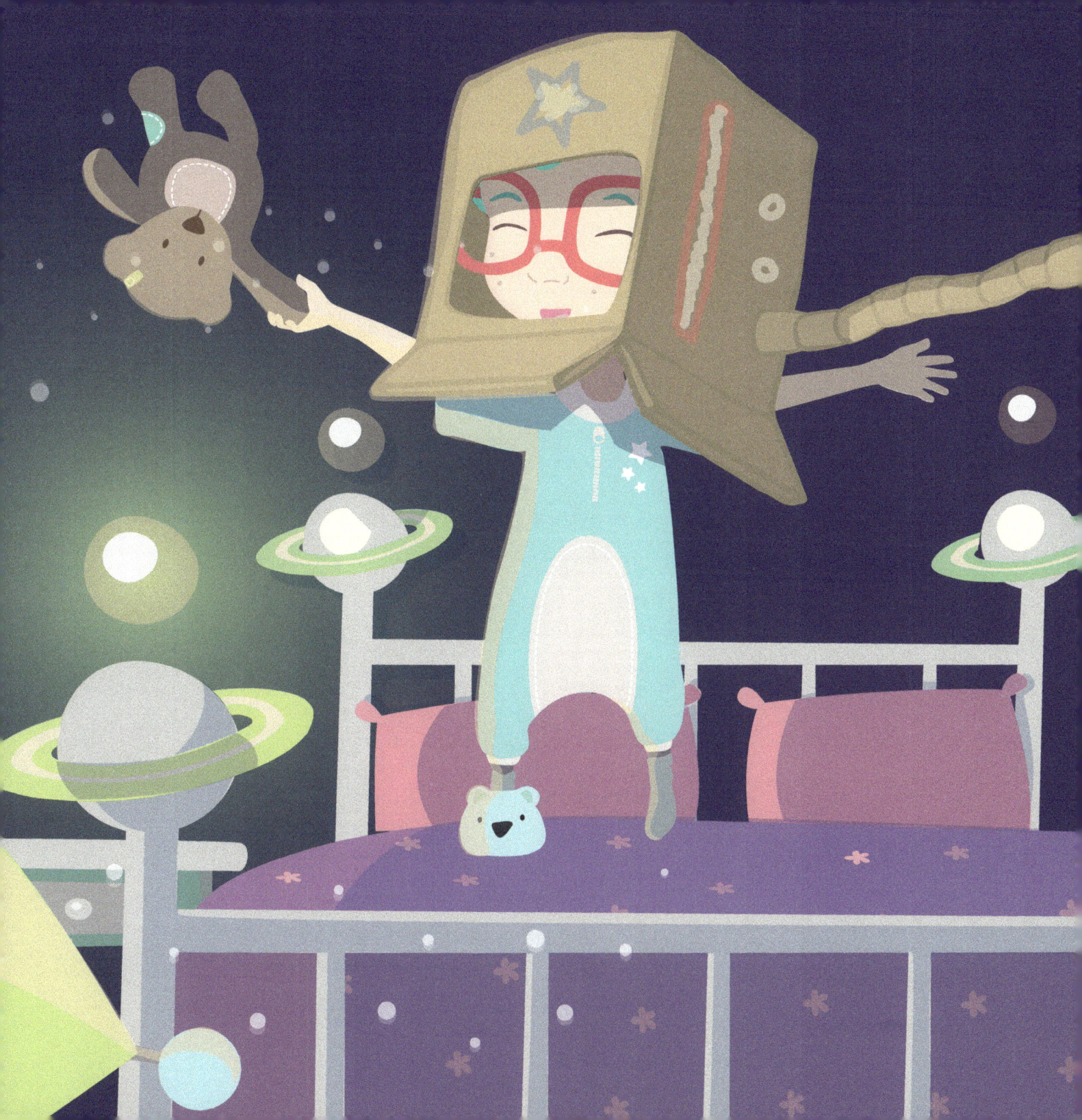

– I WANT MORE, I WANT MORE, A BIT MORE…

– FINE THEN, MANY MORE KISSES.

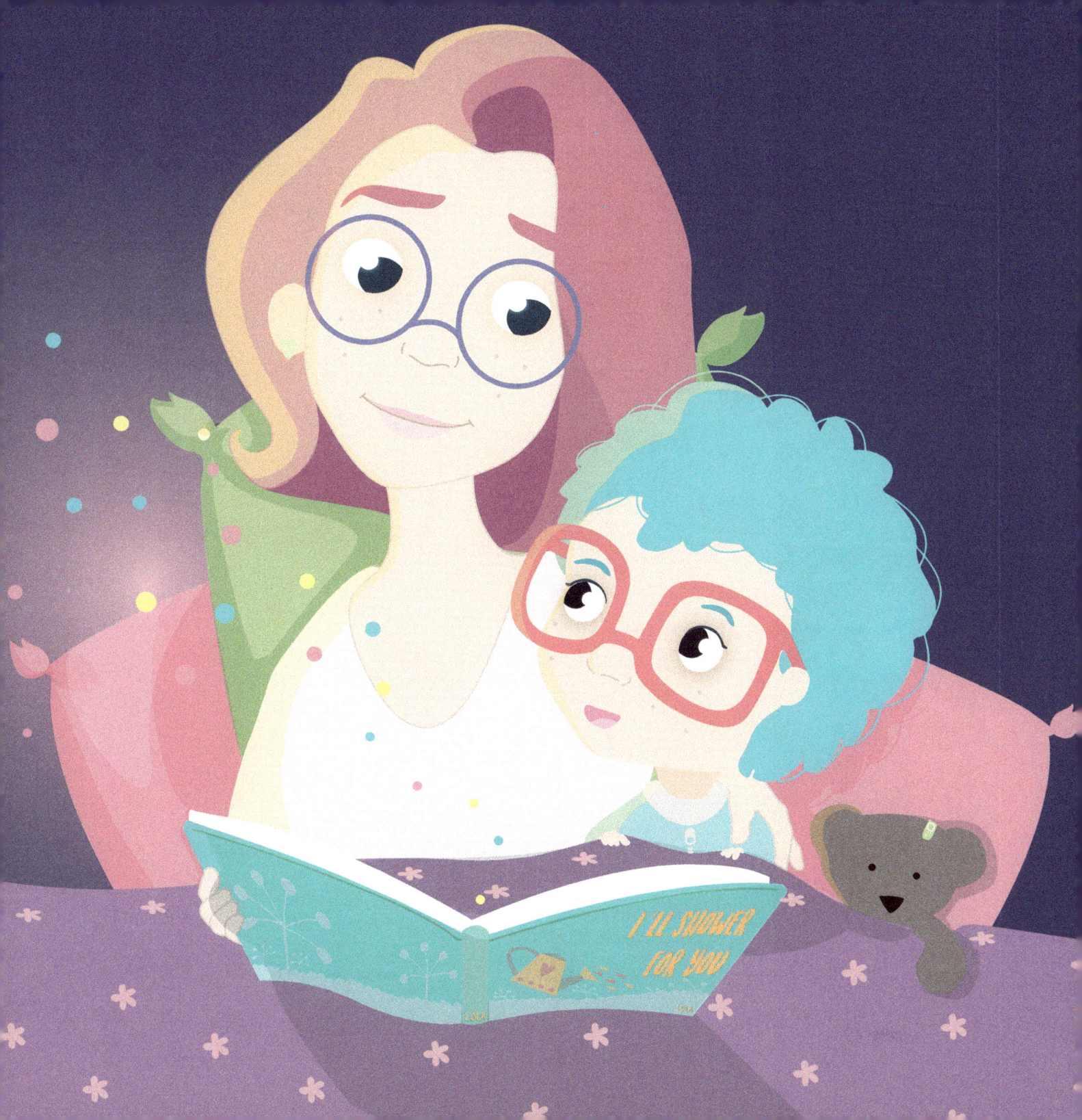

SOMETHING TERRIBLE HAS HAPPENED,
THE CHILD'S MIND AND HEART ARE HELD HOSTAGE.

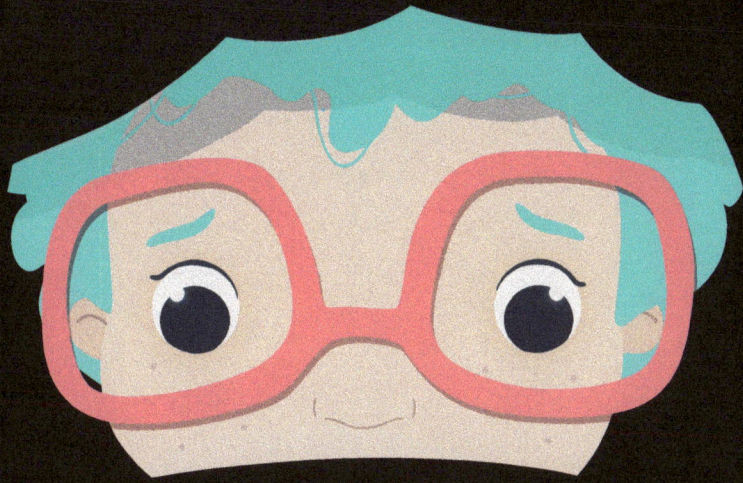

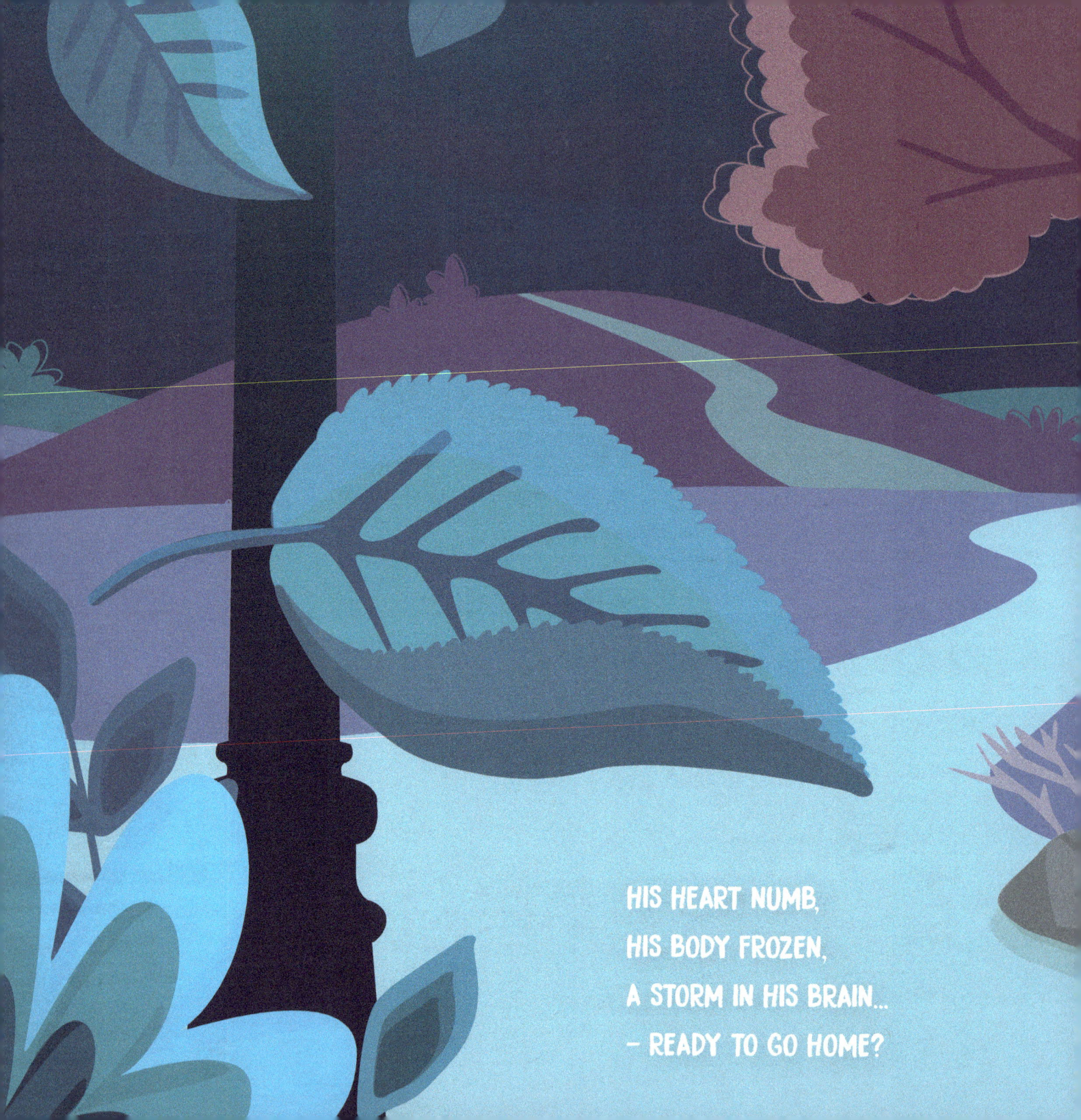

HIS HEART NUMB,
HIS BODY FROZEN,
A STORM IN HIS BRAIN...
– READY TO GO HOME?

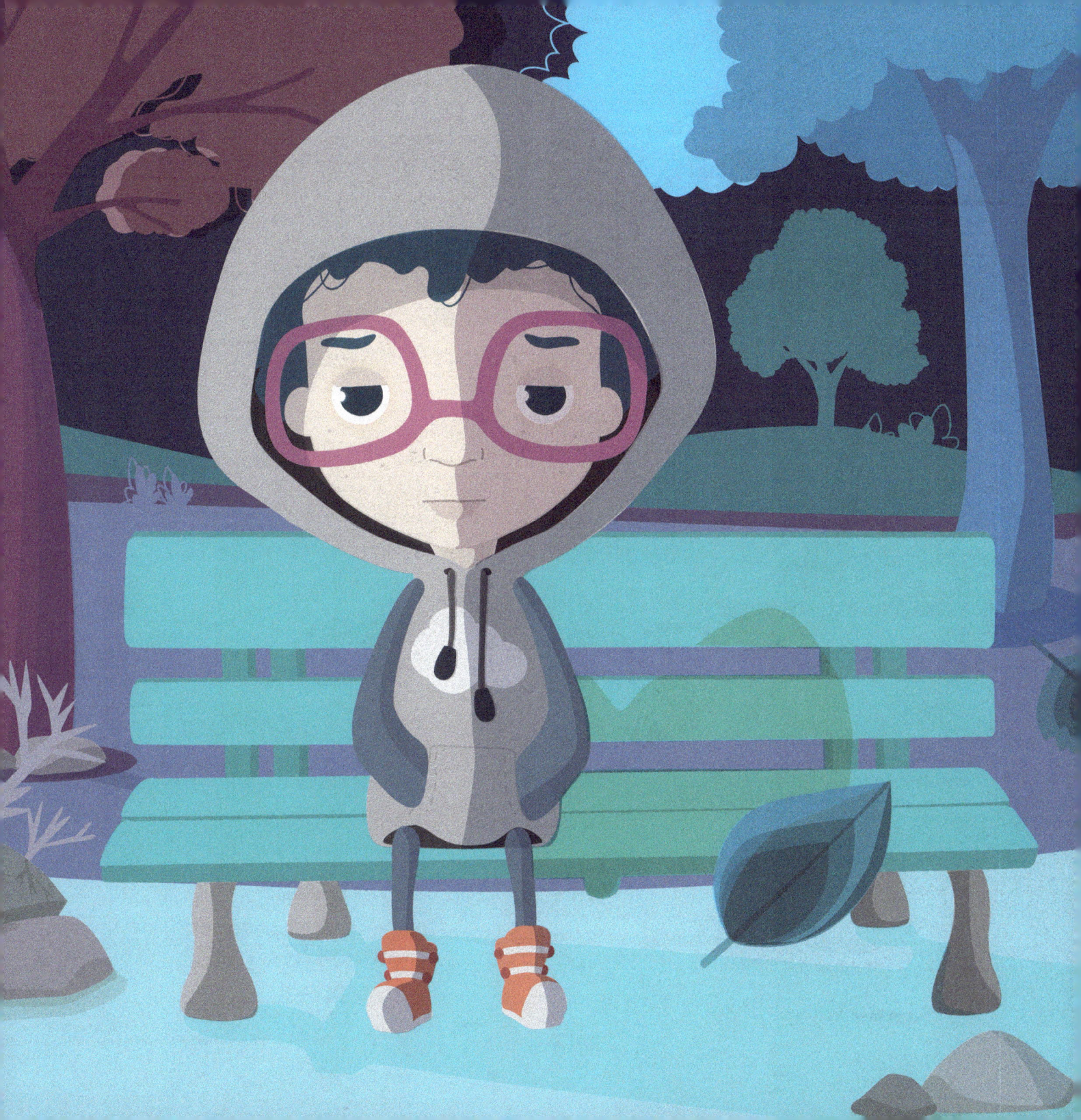

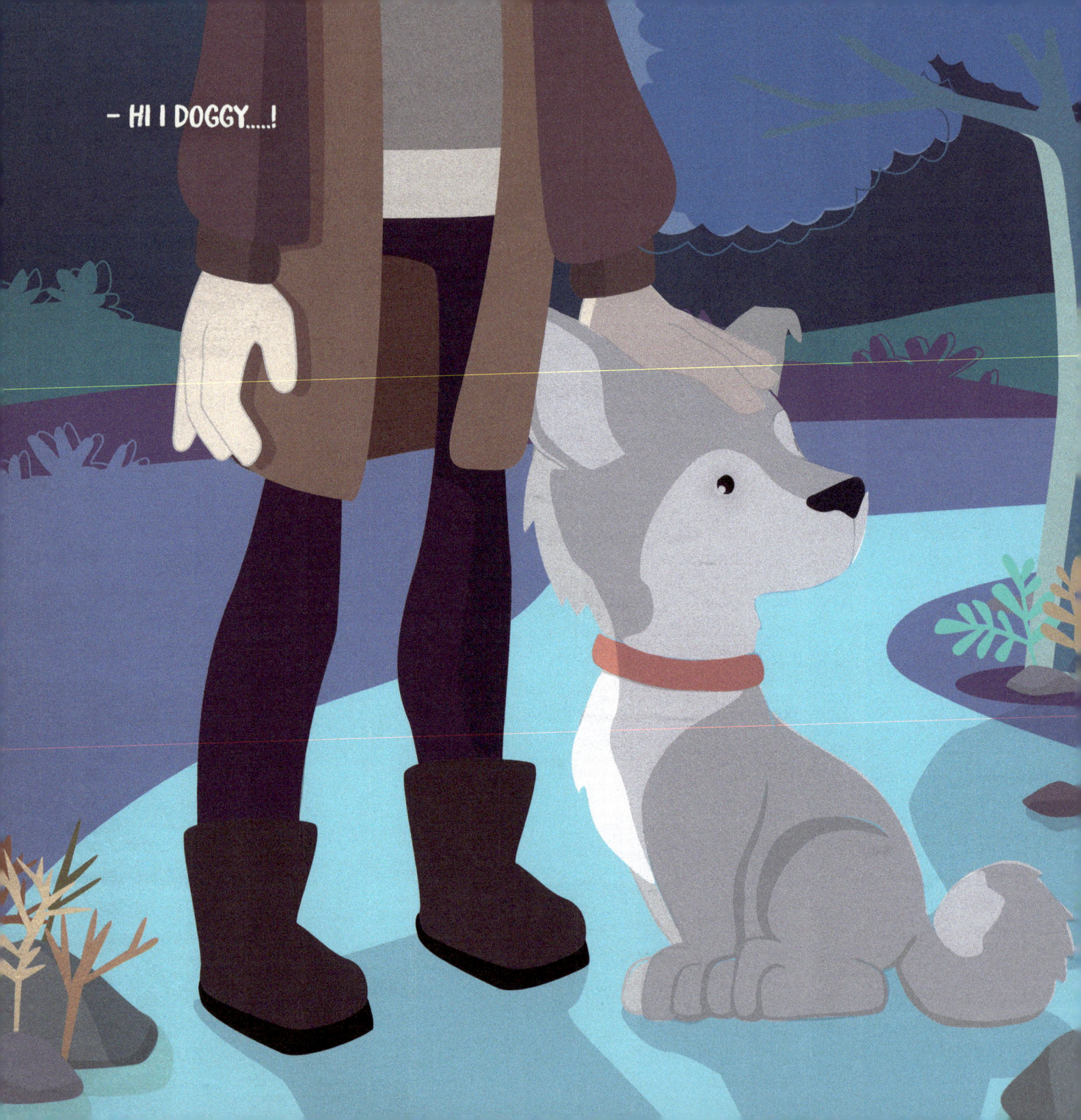

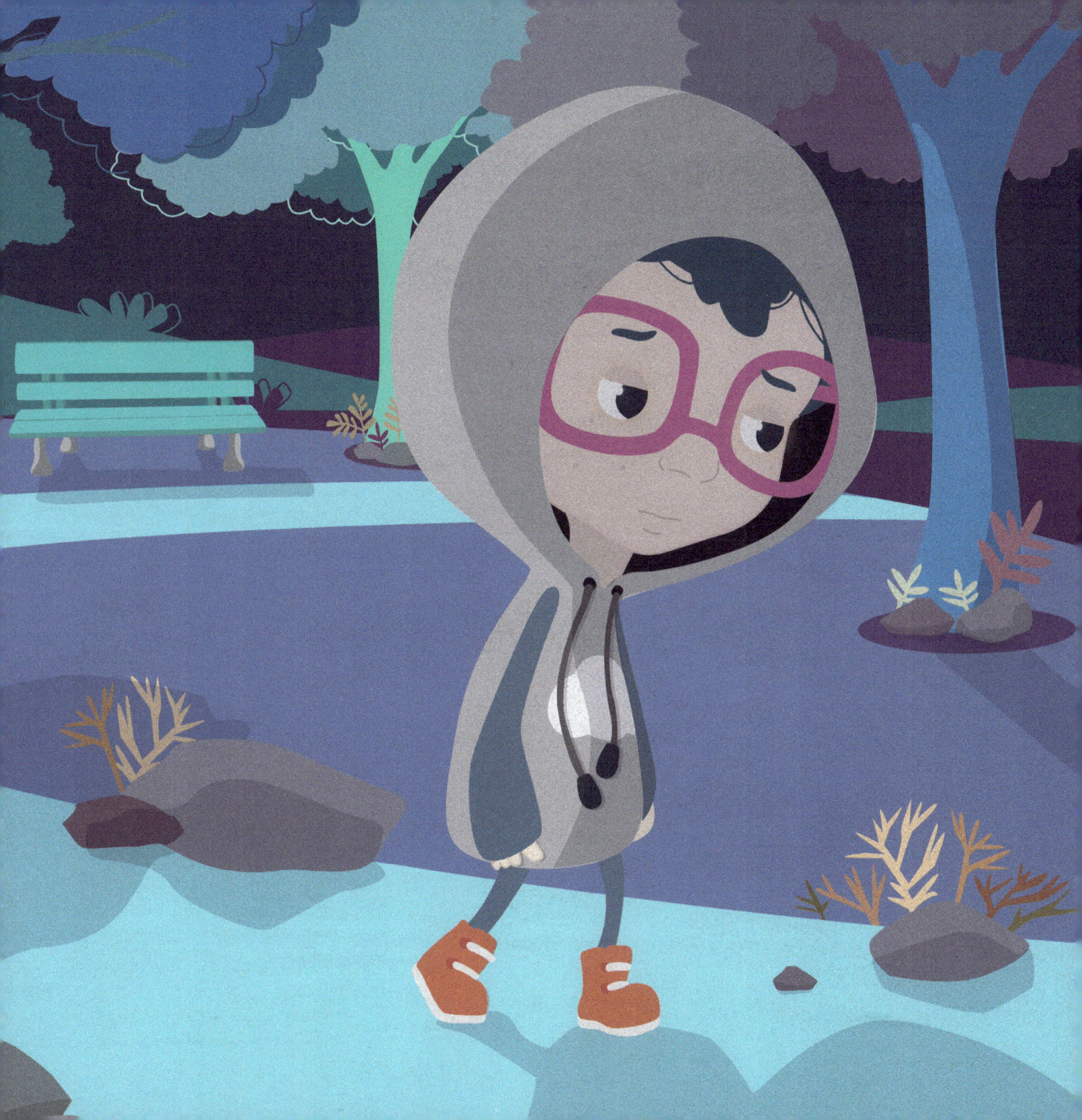

TIME FOR BED

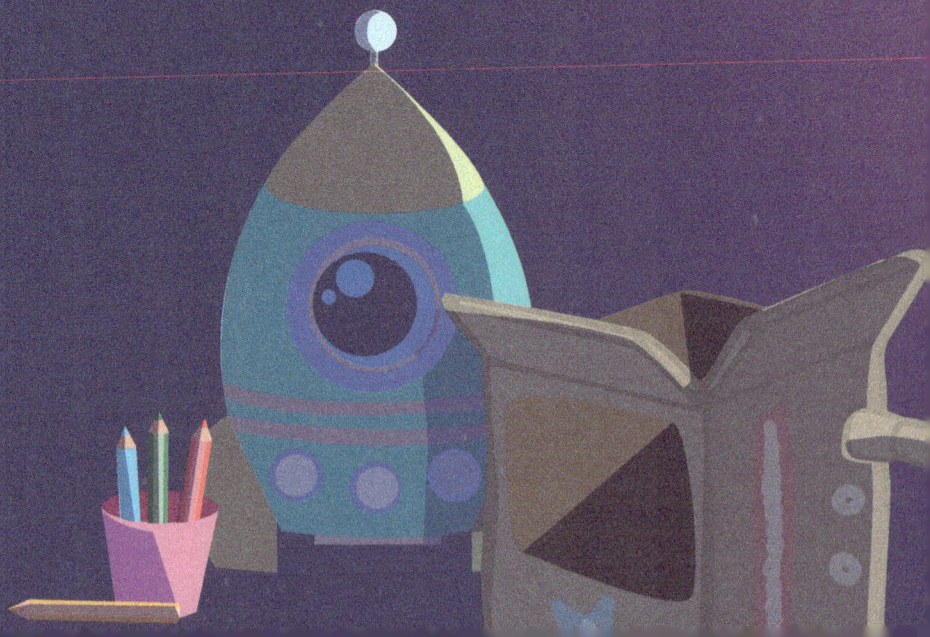

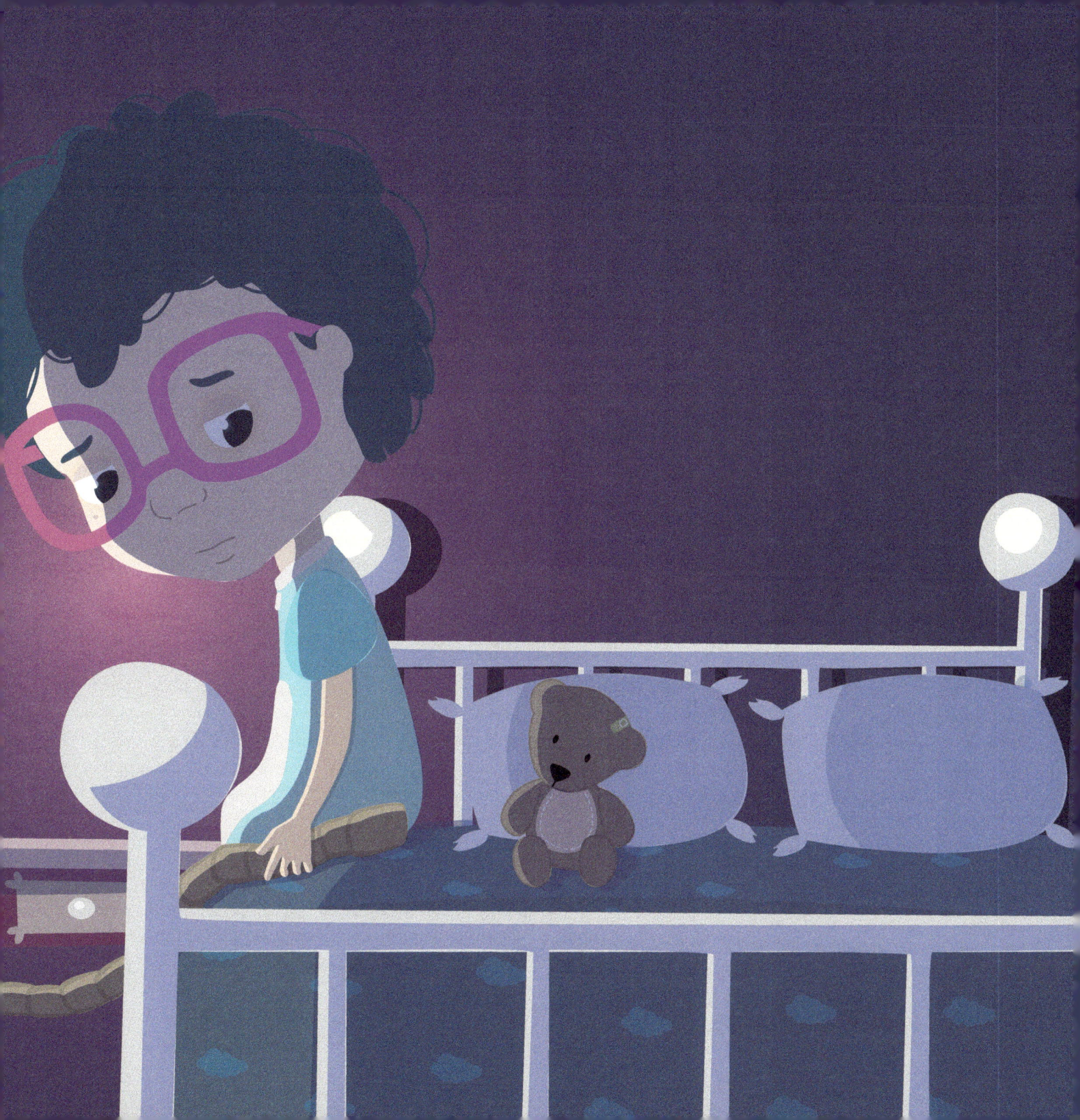

— DON'T BE AFRAID, I'M HERE WITH YOU.

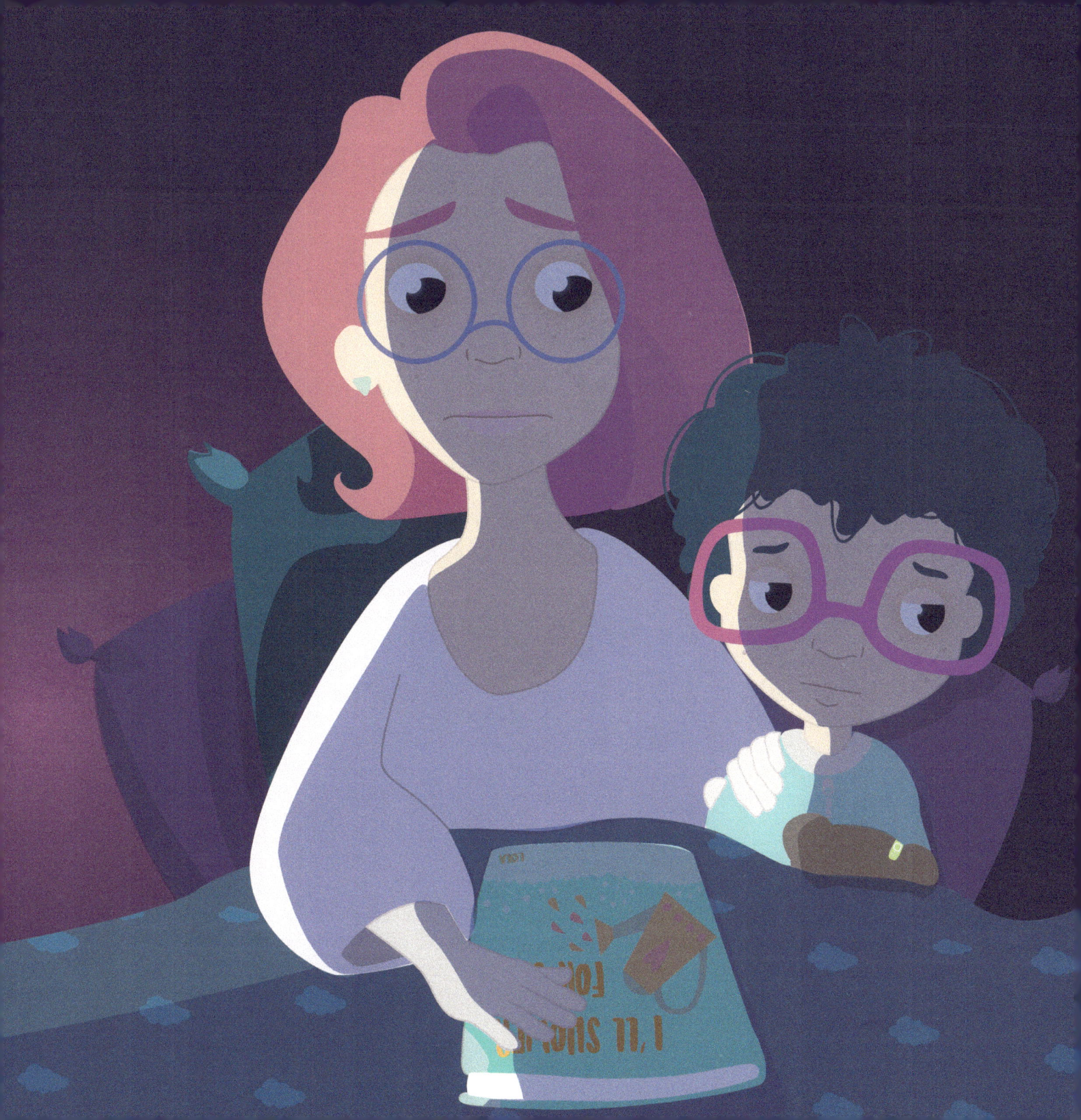

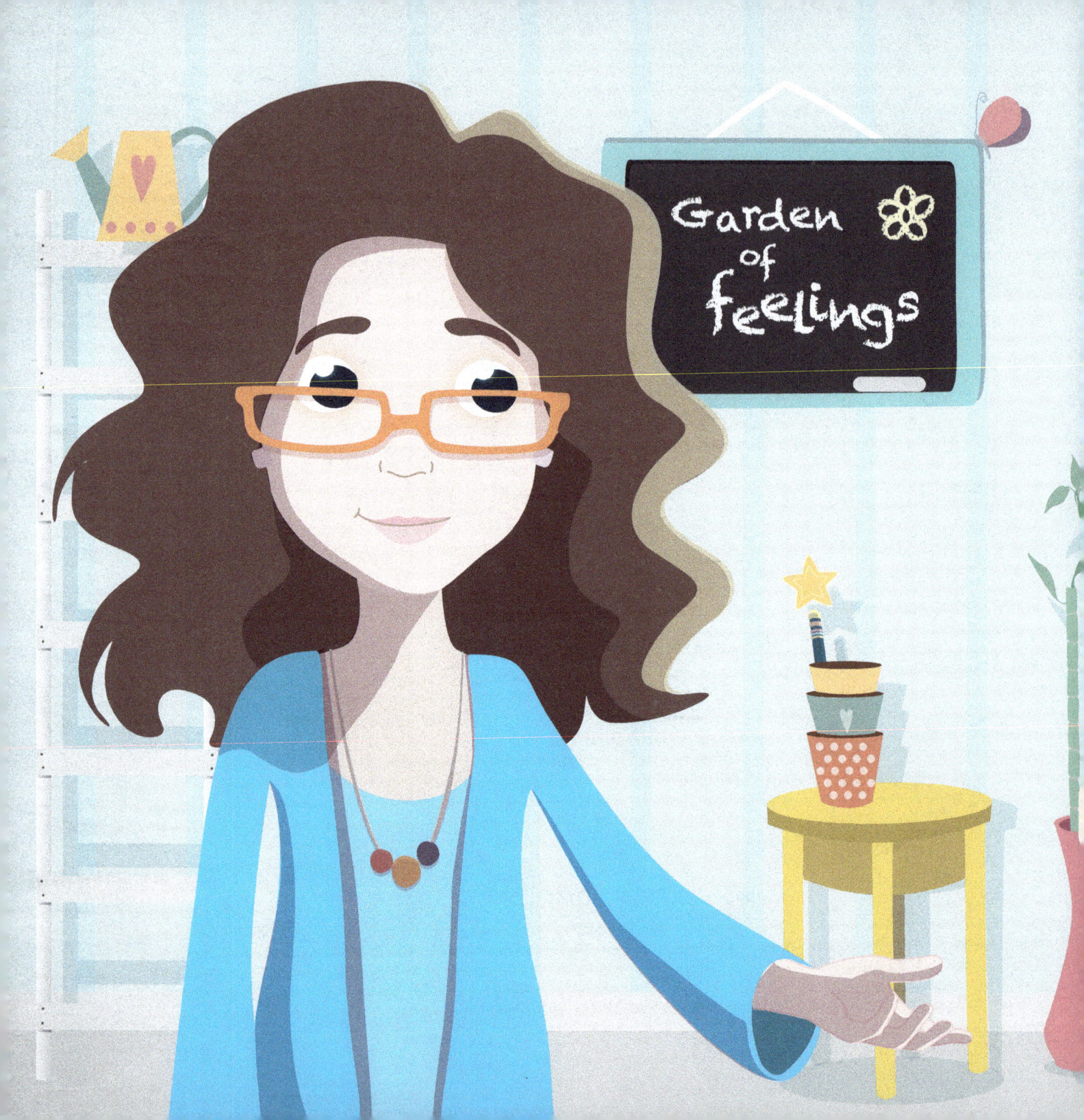

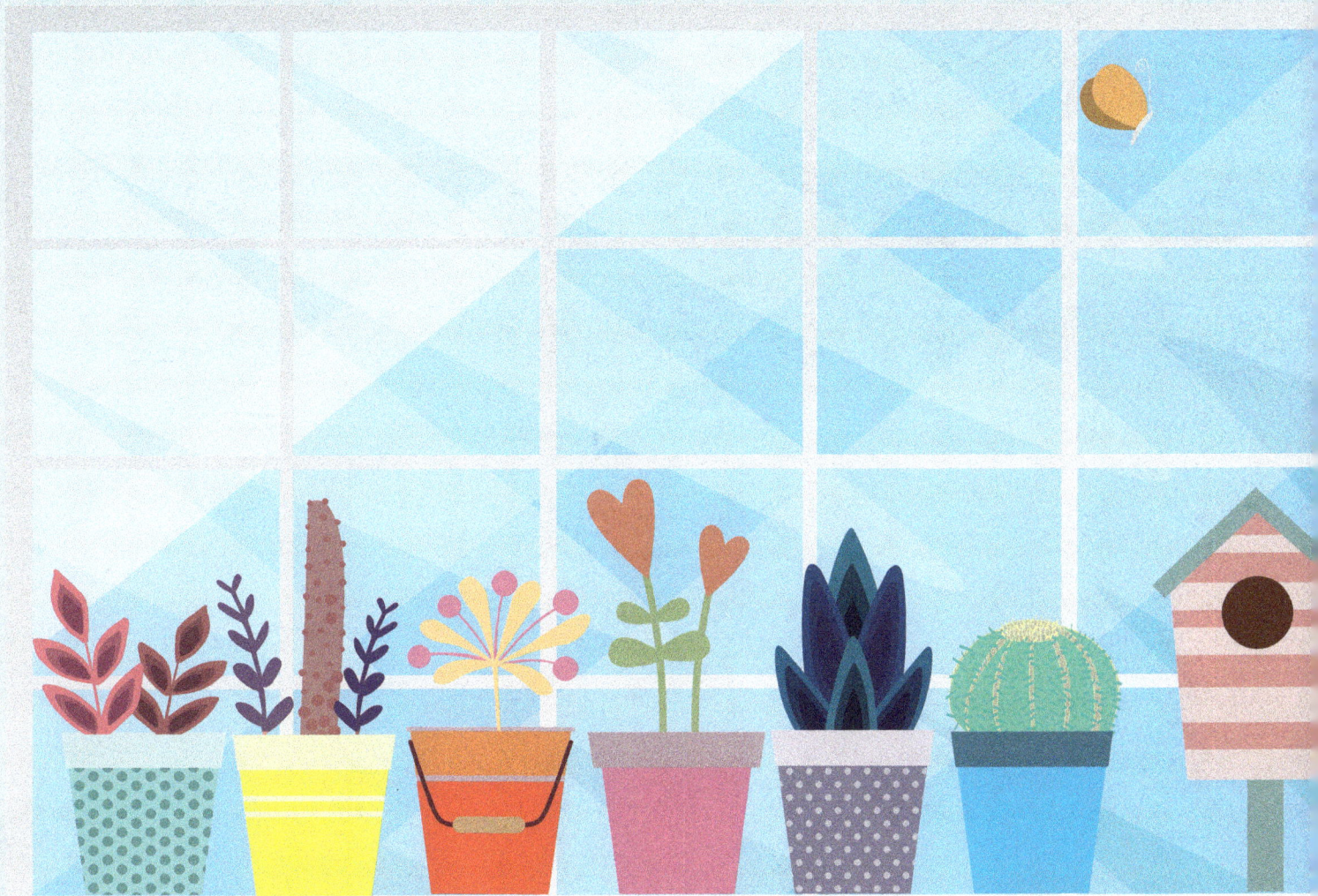

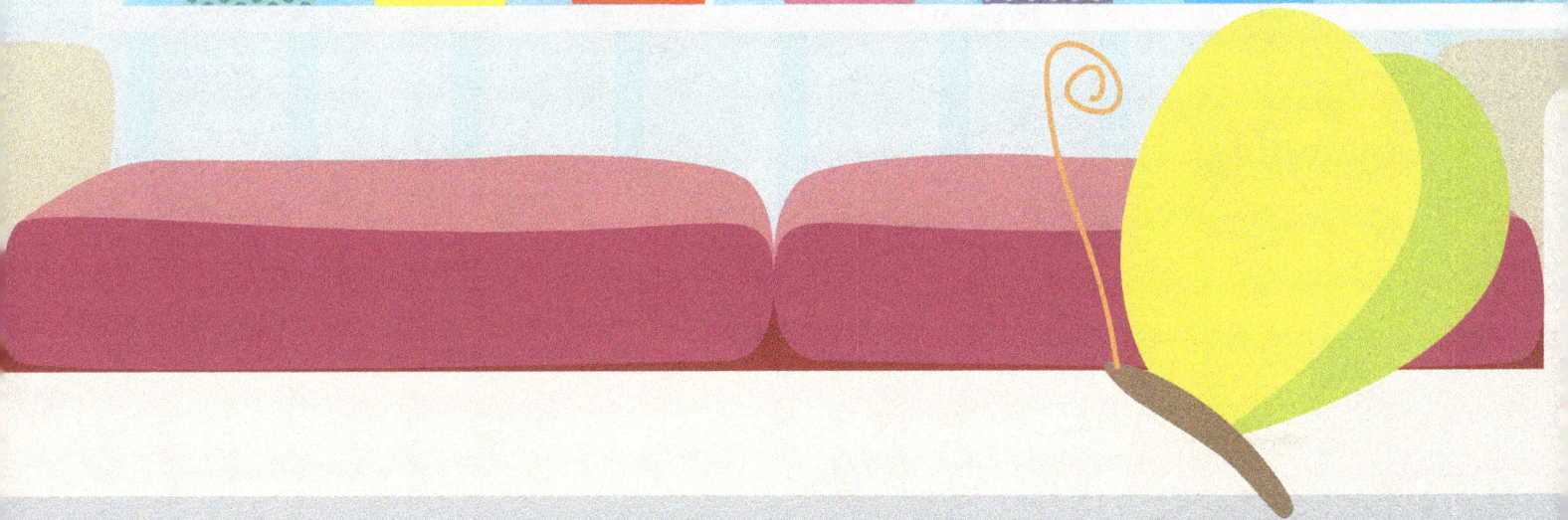

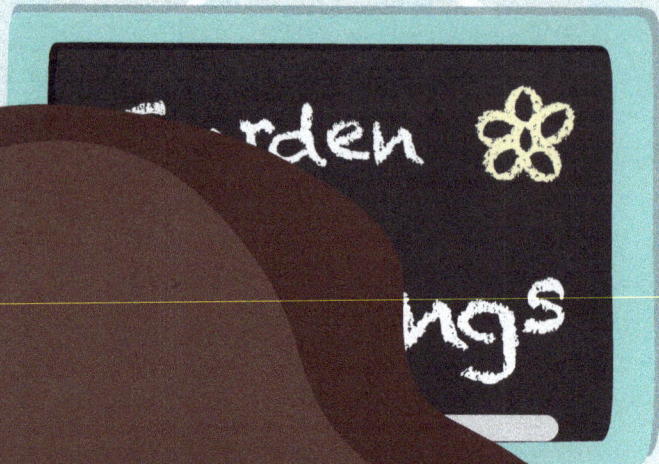

- LOOK WHERE YOU ARE AND WHO ARE WITH YOU... HERE AND NOW, YOU ARE SAFE.

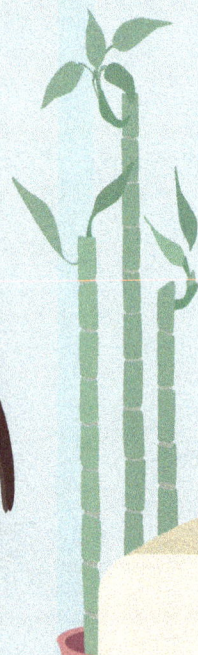

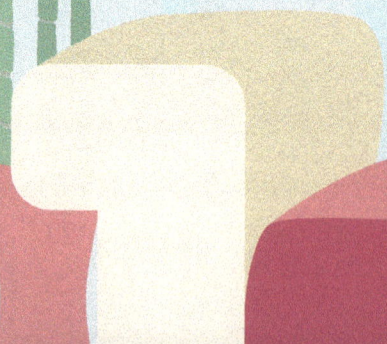

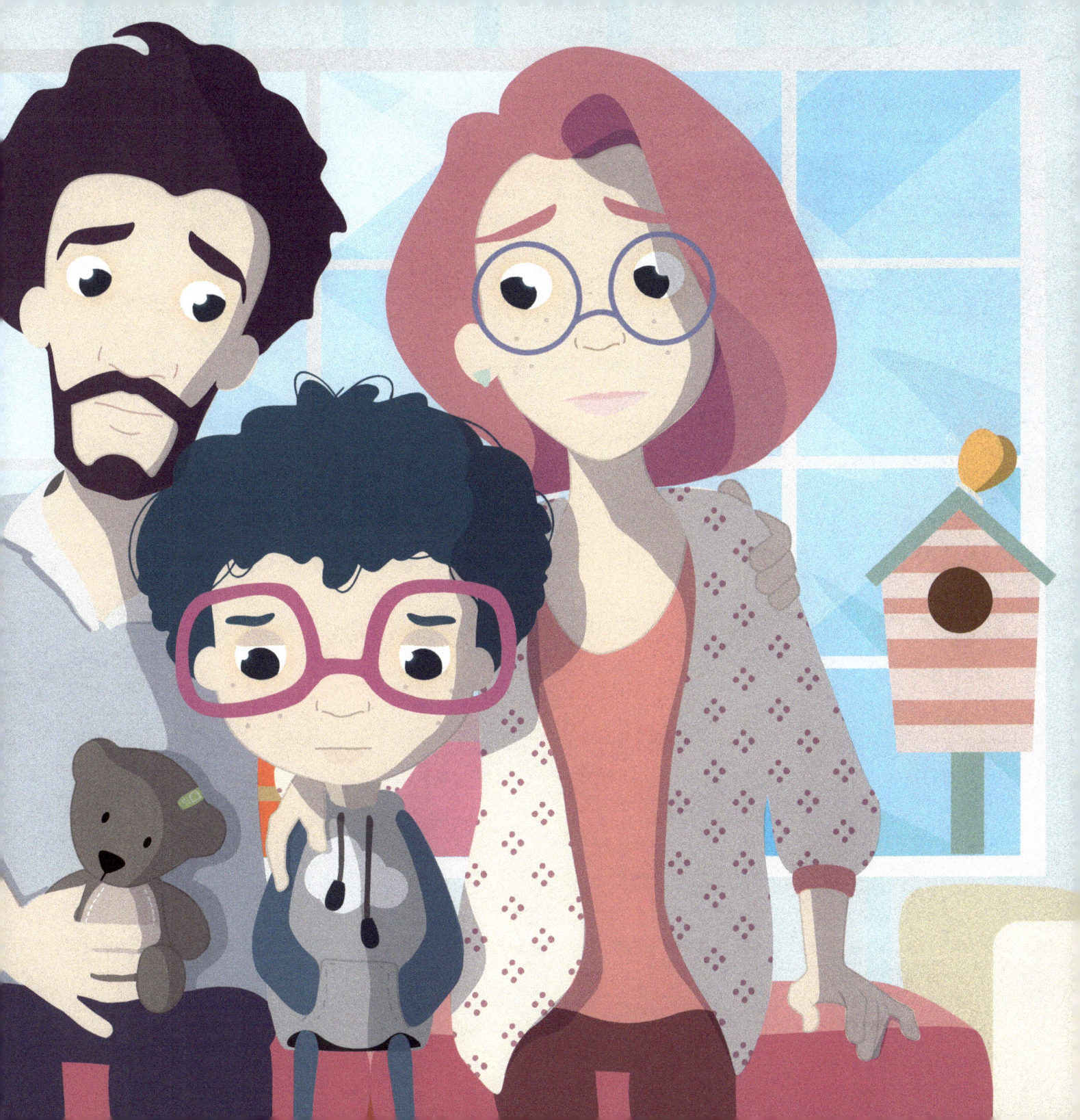

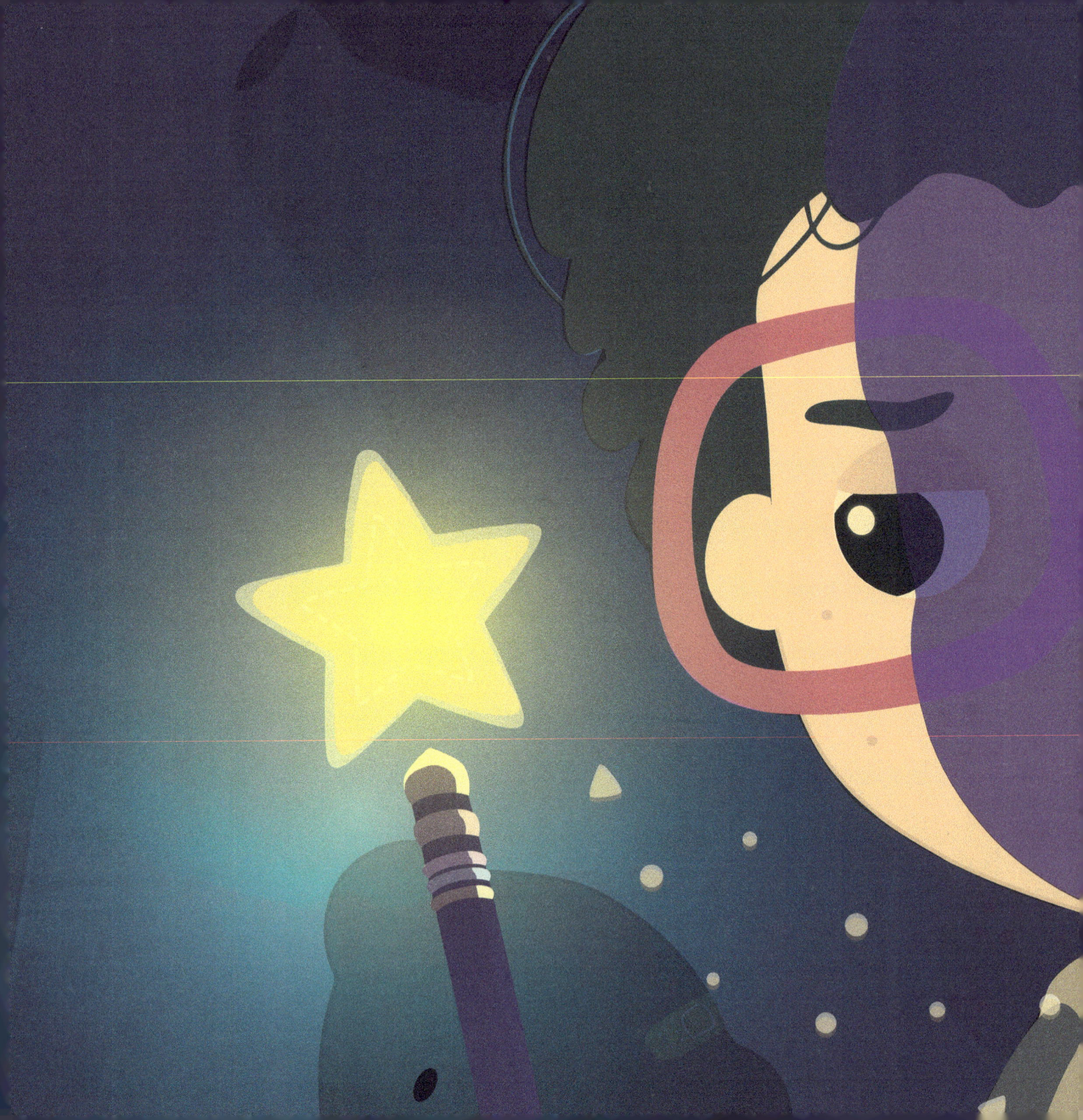

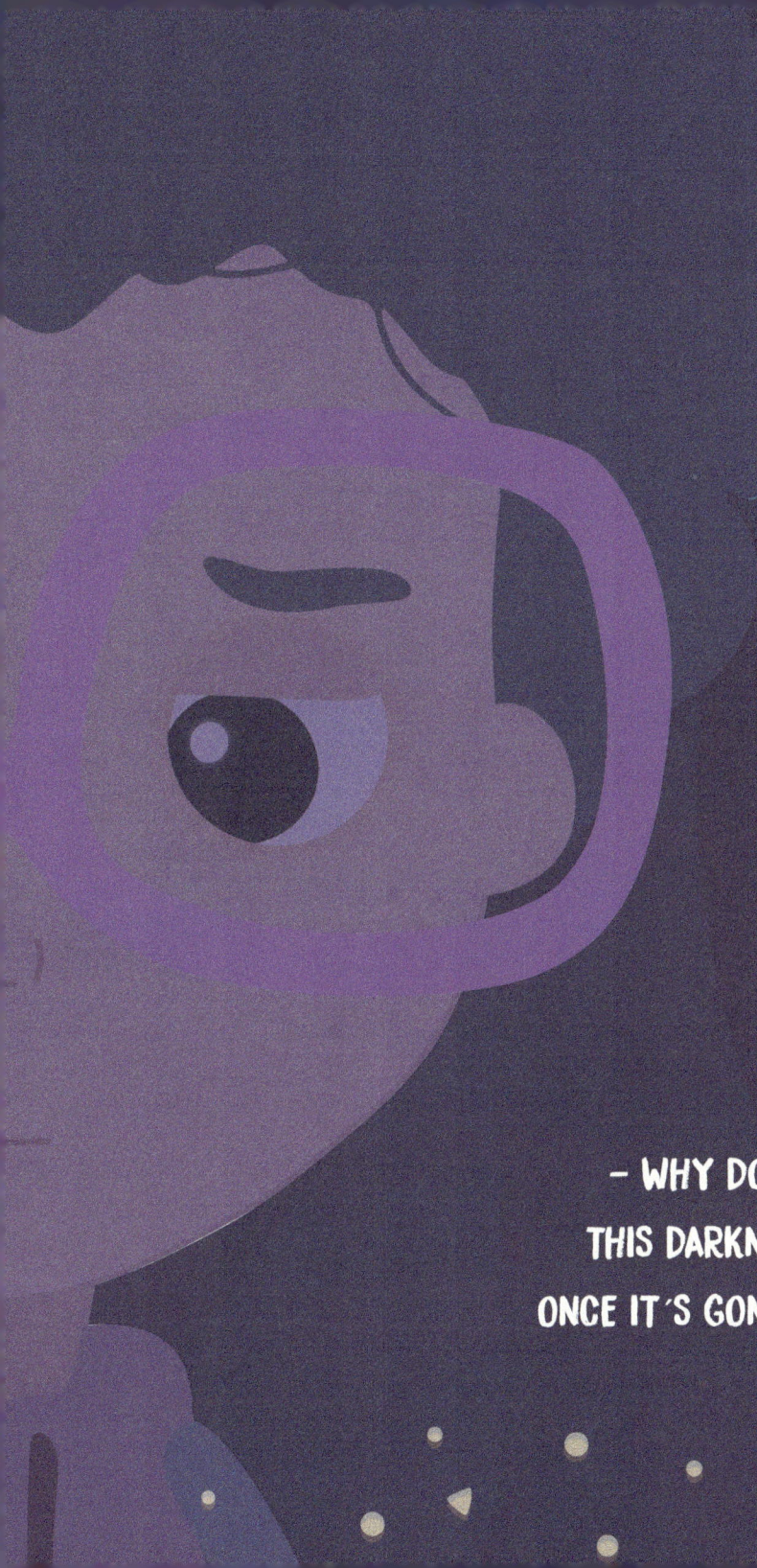

– WHY DON'T WE TRY AND TOUCH
THIS DARKNESS TO SEE IF IT GOES AWAY?
ONCE IT'S GONE, YOU MAY FEEL LIKE PLAYING AGAIN.

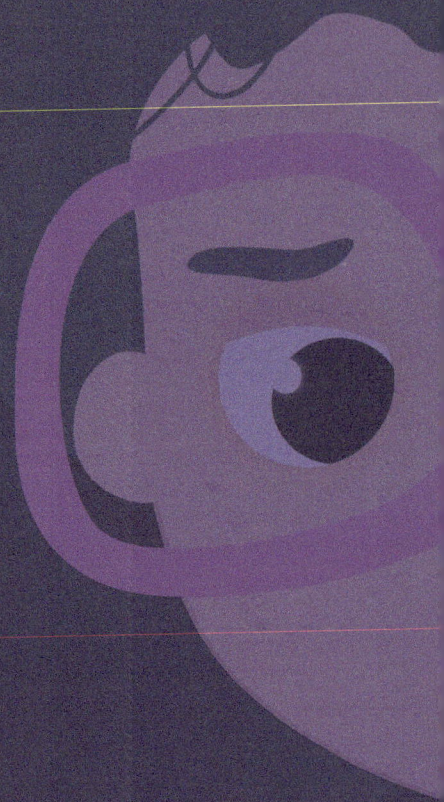
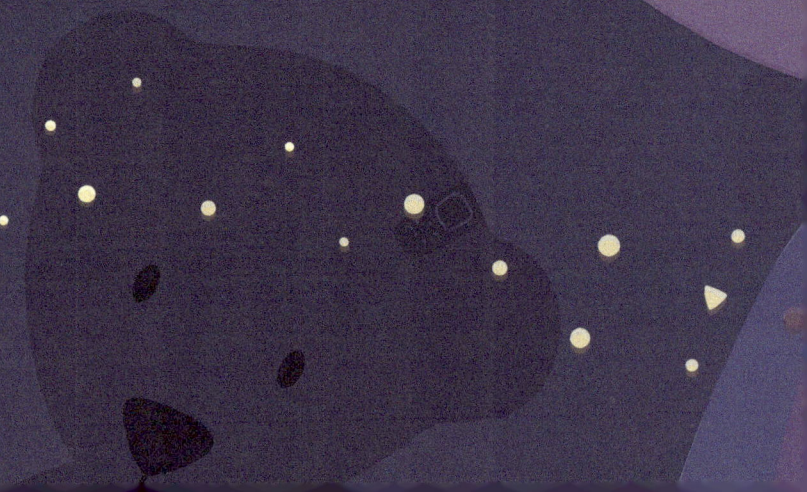

— KEEP IT UP.

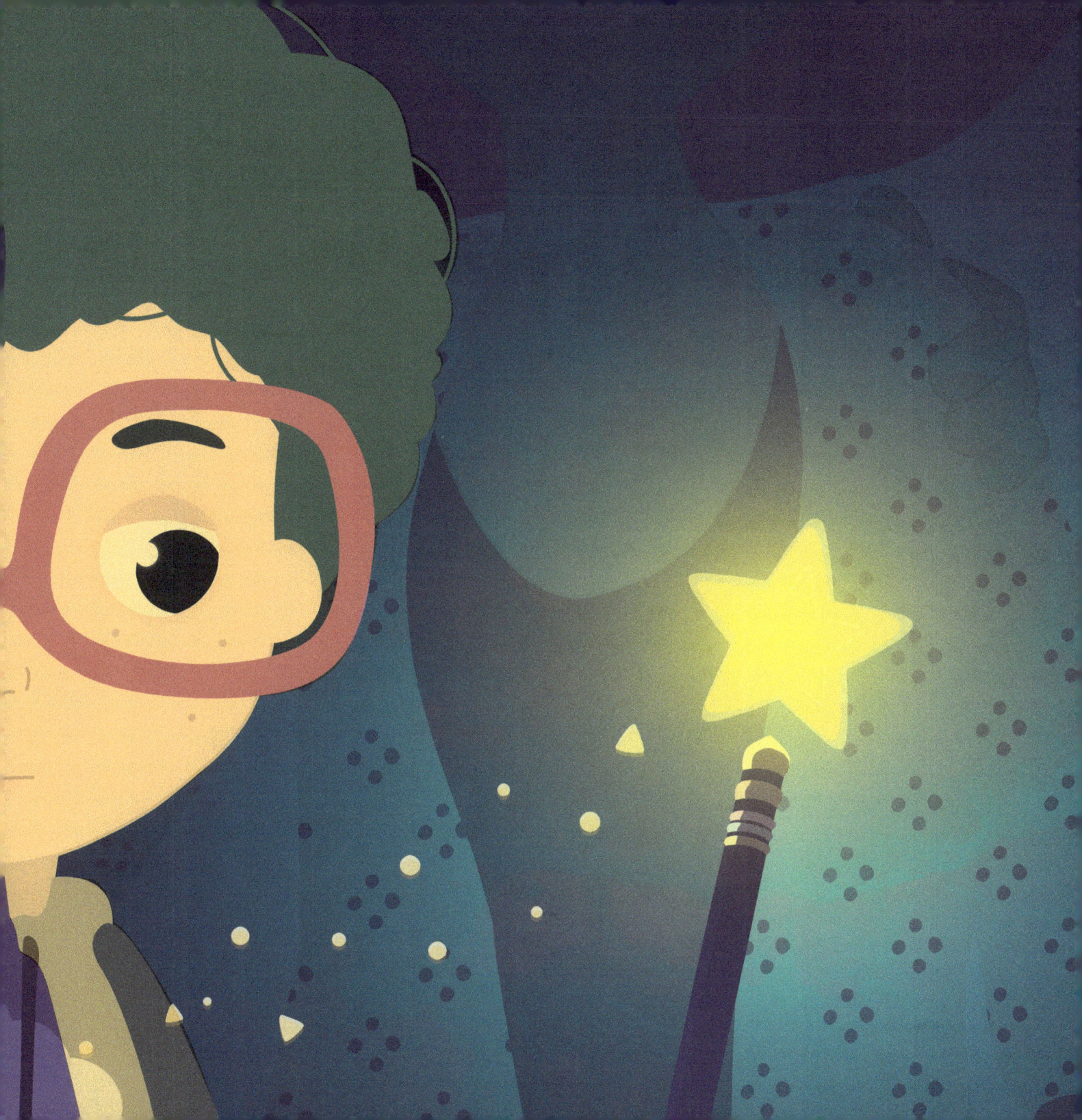

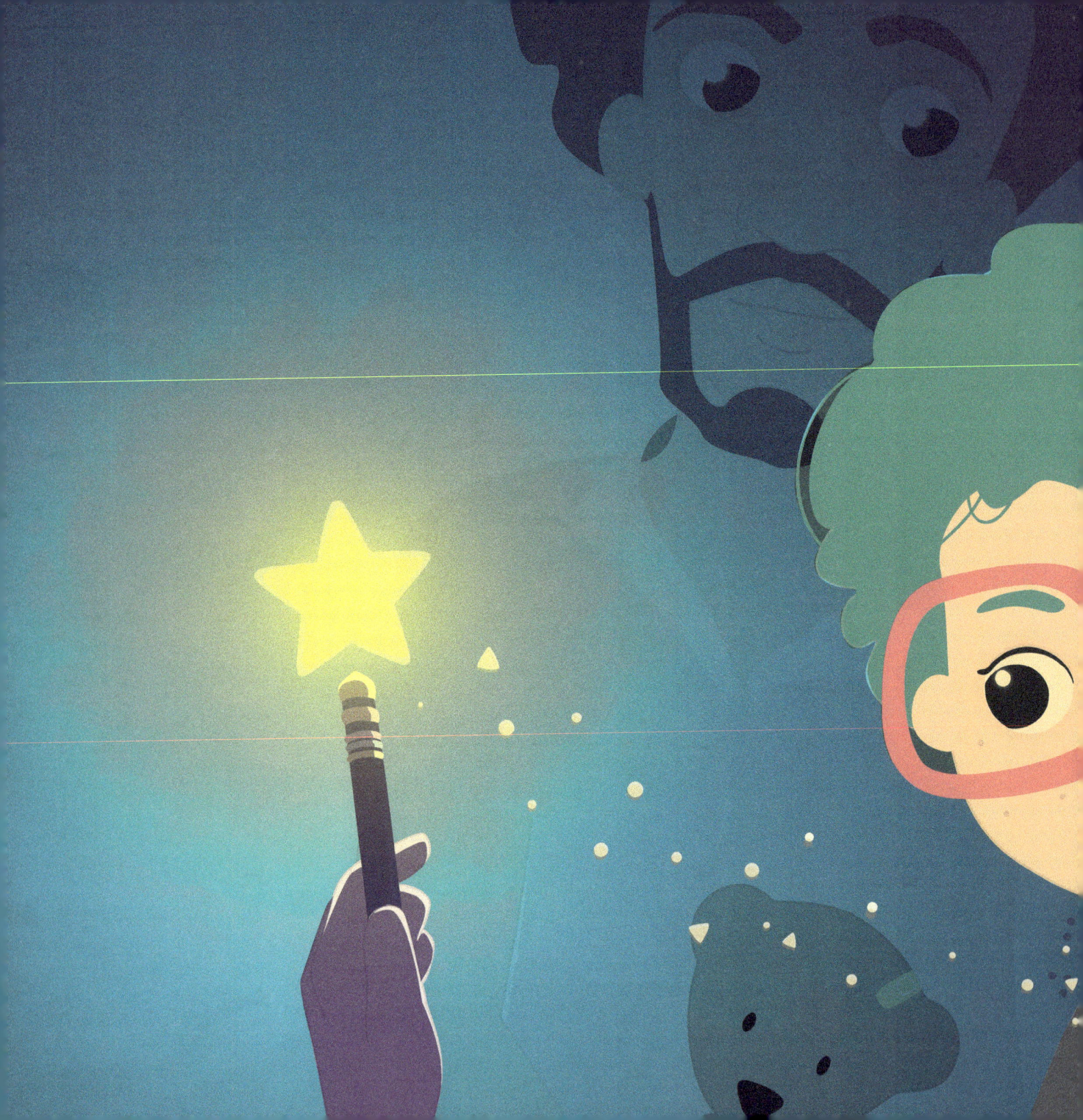

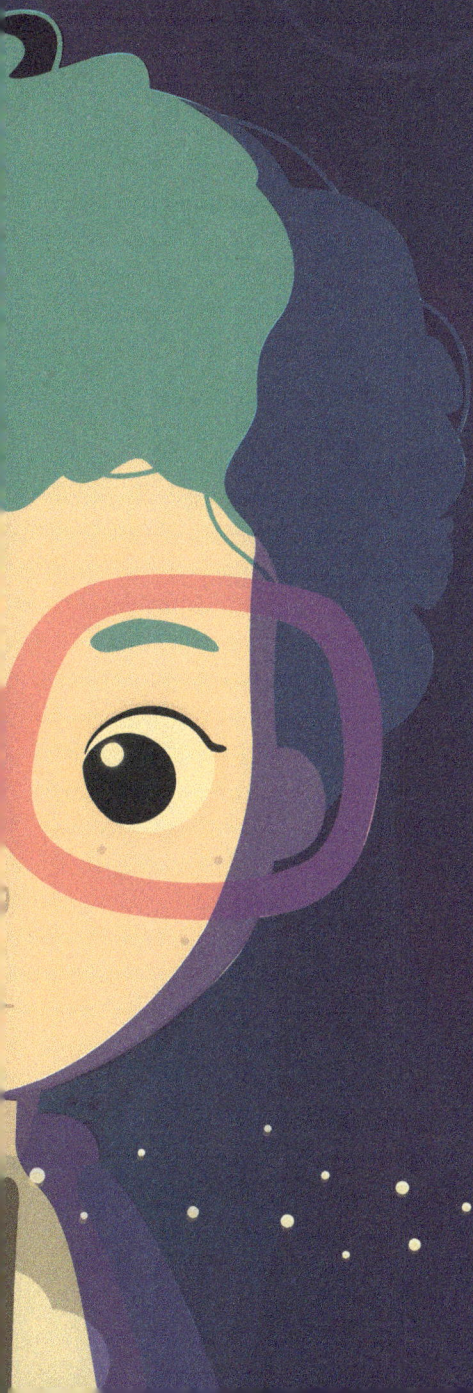

— KEEP IT UP.

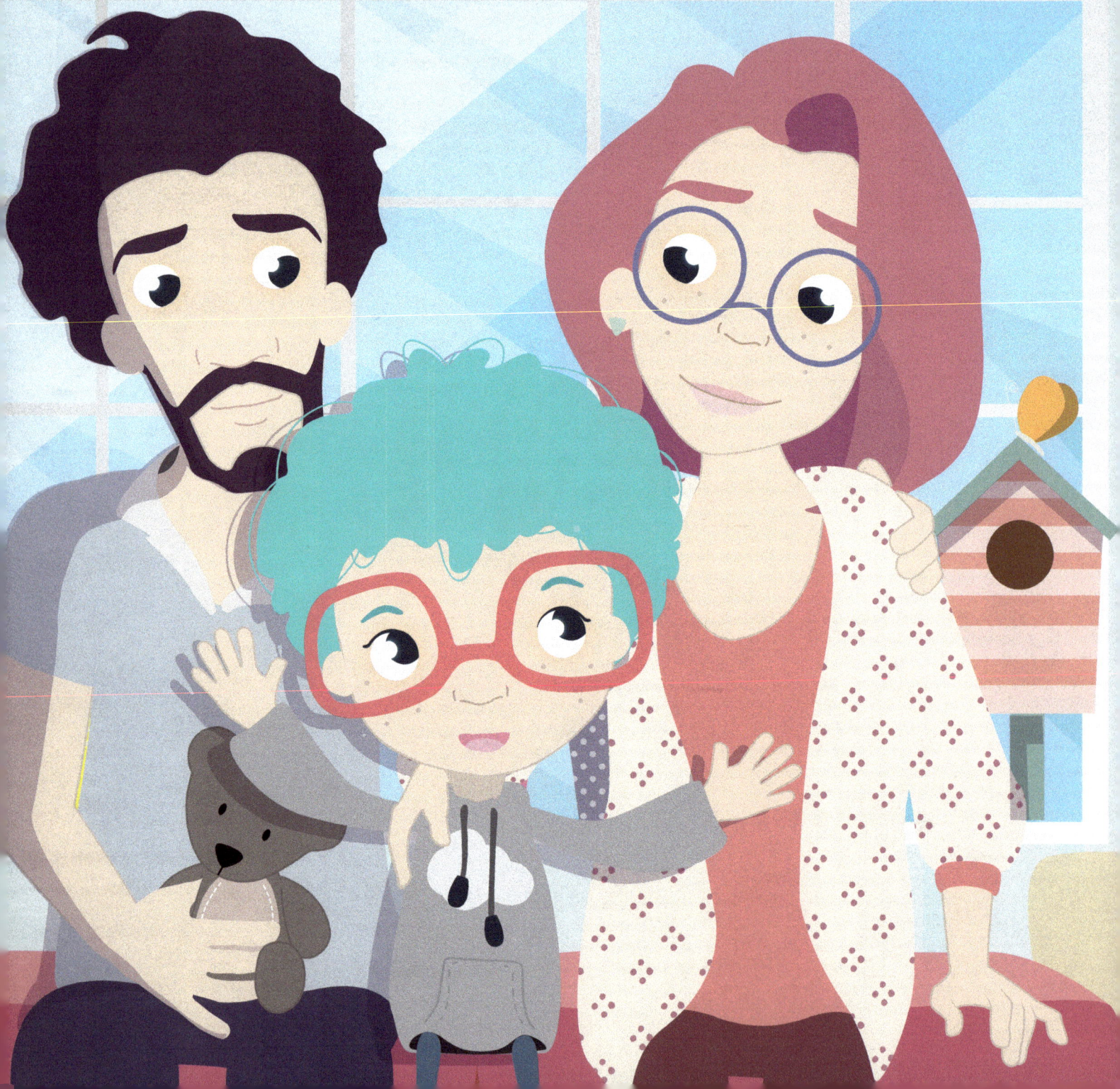

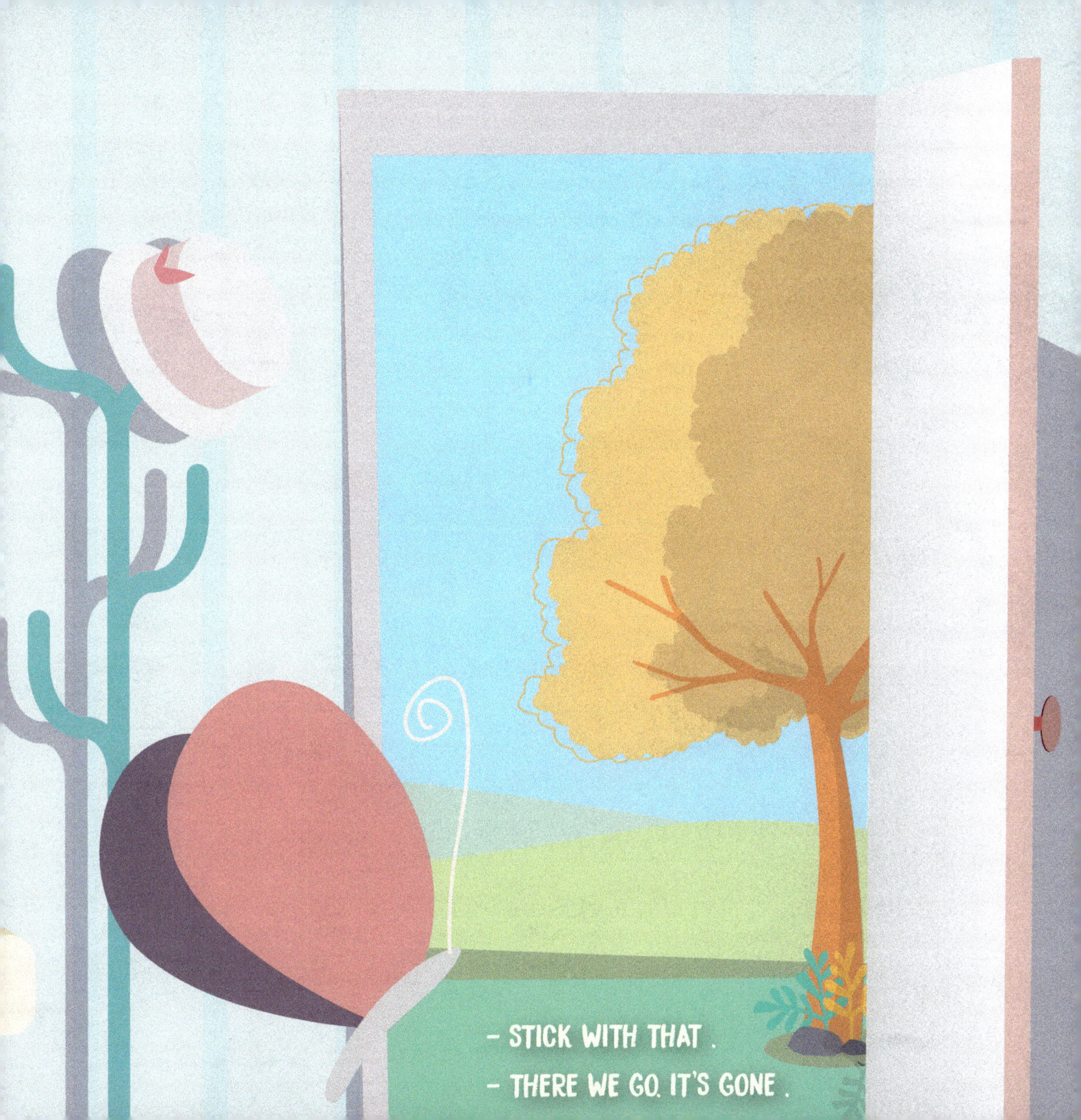

- STICK WITH THAT .
- THERE WE GO. IT'S GONE .

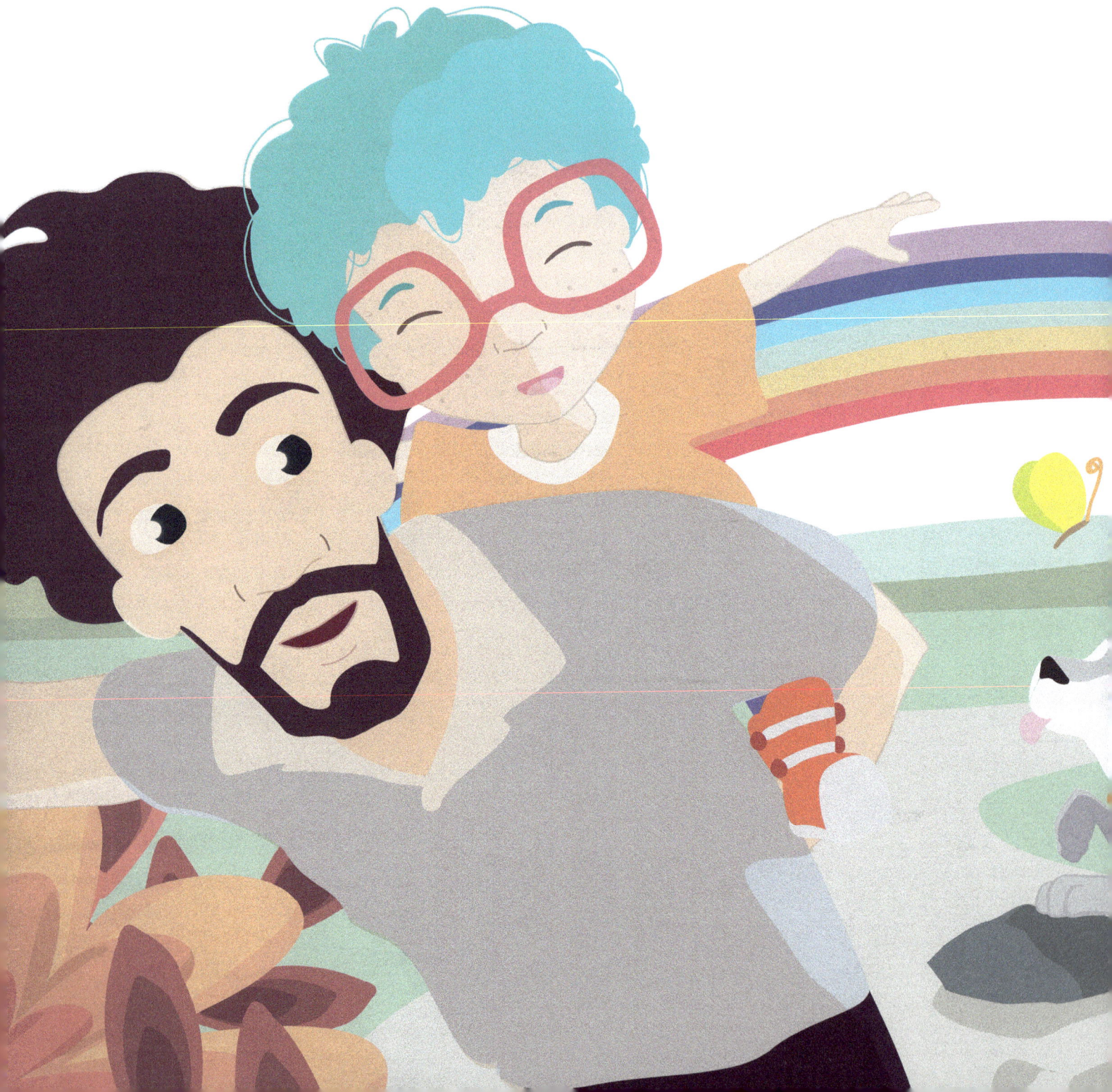

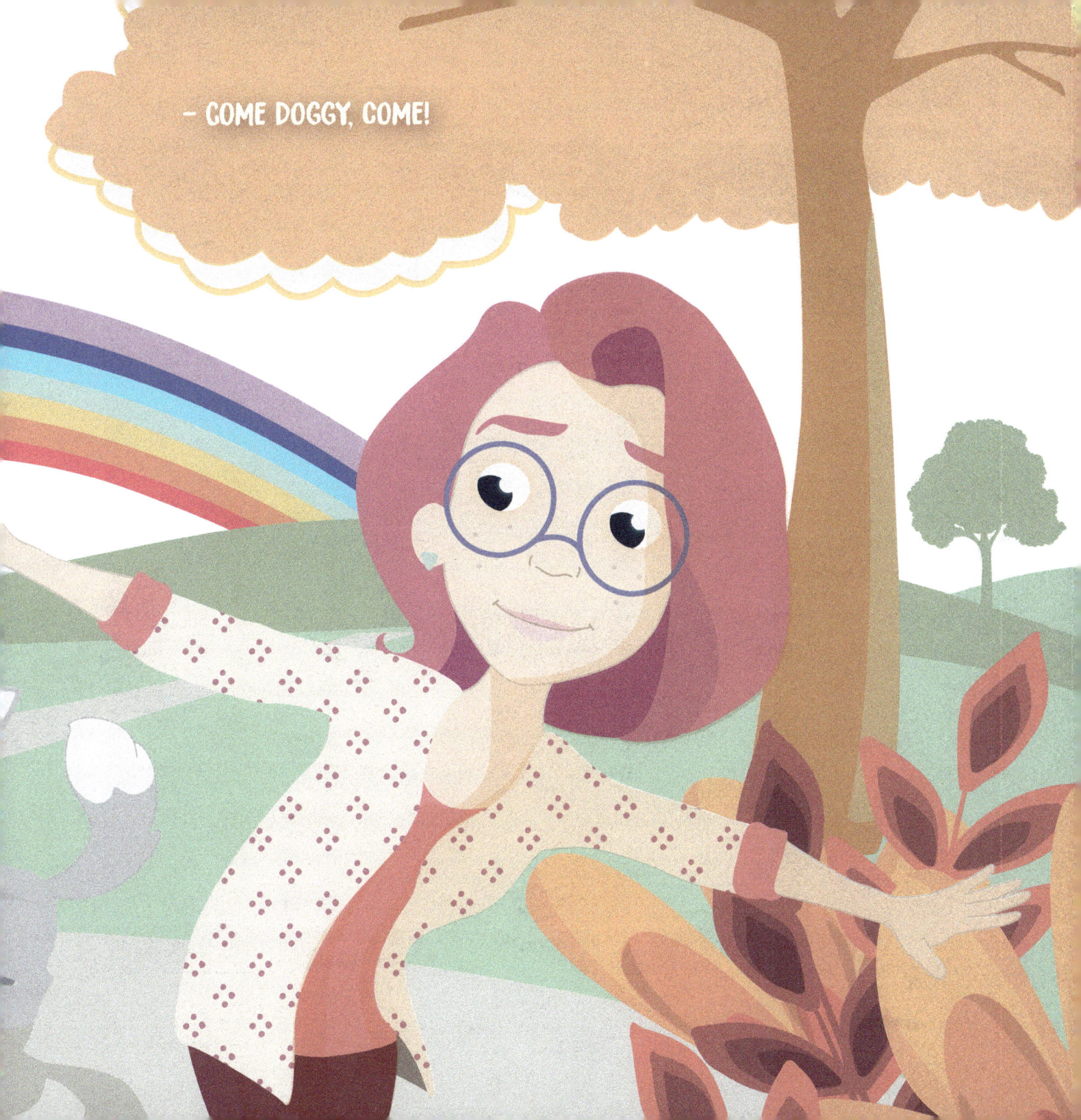

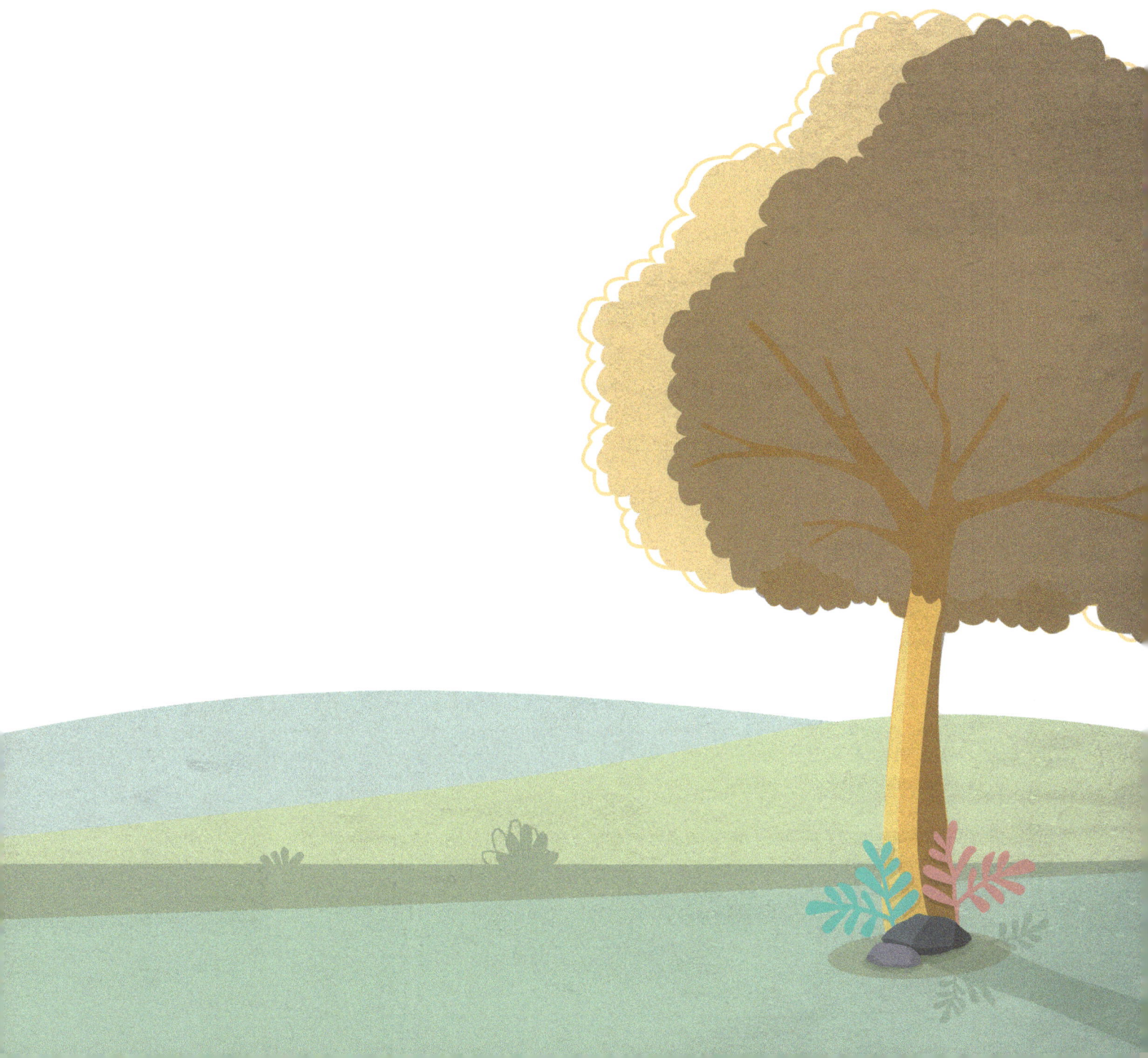

HOW TO EXPLAIN EMDR TO CHILDREN?

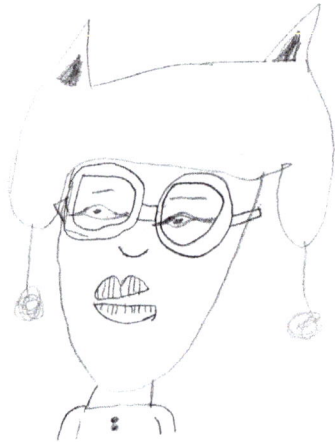

Allow me to explain what EMDR is and how it works. This series of letters indicates that stimulating Eye Movement helps us to Digest elements that have caused us suffering. This includes topics which we are unable to share or express, whether this is because we have forgotten them, do not know how to share them, or because reflecting upon them scares us greatly.

Through the dance of the eyes, the discomfort, the hidden fear in the body enclosed within the heart, huddled in the depths of our thoughts, diminishes and can even disappear. We can recover the joy, security, the desire to play, to kiss and to embrace. These Regained desires are felt in the body, the gut, the heart and in the mind.

There are burdensome and unpleasant sensations that rob the body of energy or inhibit us from feeling. They might be emotions of sadness or pain that disturb our hearts and chests, as well as dark and cloudy thoughts. We might believe that we are in danger, that something terrible is going to happen, or that we are alone and cannot turn to anyone. Such thoughts all dissolve and disappear as our eyes dance, moving in fits and starts.

You will ask yourself "Why do our eyes need to move and dance?" The answer is quite simple.

Every night, once we enter a phase of sleep known as REM (rapid eye movement), our eyes dance. Some dance to Rock n' Roll, others to flamenco or samba, depending on their rhythm and passion. Our eyes followed this dance, this rhythm, even when we were safely nestled in our mother's womb. As they jump and dance, our eyes organize, link and sort out everything that we have seen throughout the day, including both the good and not so good experiences, and the darkness clears up. As a result, our memories and experiences are ordered, and we can navigate through them and reflect upon them without feeling bad.

When a psychologist asks you to let your eyes dance during the day, they want to help you organize the broken pieces of the painful experiences. They want to help you organize experiences that have remained detached, hidden or buried within the pain of your body, mind and heart, so as to create a shining star, without pain, that allows you to regain the desire to live with enthusiasm.

For this reason, I present you with this children's book How can I get out of here?

This is the story of a boy, a girl, any child who lives, plays, laughs and enjoys life until, one day, something happens. That something can be many different things, different for each child, who afterwards stops laughing, playing and jumping, and who finds that everything turns grey.

Fortunately, someone invites their eyes to dance. And as the eyes move, jump and dart around, all those dark clouds fade away. All those messy fragments fall into line and, as a result, the child regains the vital energy, as well as the glimmer in their eyes and their peace of mind. They can continue their journey through life, growing up full of curiosity and vitality.

If something bad happened in your life and the pain is still with you, and even if you have grown accustomed to this pain, I invite you to let your eyes dance.

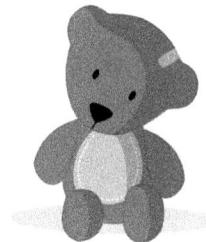

FOR PARENTS, PSYCHOTHERAPISTS AND TEACHERS

A SHORT EXPLANATION OF CHILD EMDR THERAPY

Our childhood is one of the most decisive periods in our lives, and from it we learn about the world based on our experiences in those first few years.

These experiences are seen, felt and transmitted through attachment figures, caregivers and teachers.

Each of these figures conveys their vision of reality, a reality that is merged with our disposition, and shapes who we are.

As a result of the most decisive relationships, we create a series of mental representations of ourselves, of how valid and loved we are, of our confidence to trust others, and of how safe our world is. At this time, the brain and the nervous system are in the process of formation and development. This means that we are extremely vulnerable to emotional damage, which, if not properly tended to, can produce a negative impact throughout our development.

EMDR (Eye Movement Desensitization and Reprocessing) was developed by Dr Francine Shapiro. It is a psychotherapeutic approach which helps people heal by overcoming adversity or traumatic life experiences. EMDR therapy has been recognized by the WHO (World Health Organization) as an effective intervention in the treatment of post-traumatic stress.

EMDR therapy integrates elements from many psychological approaches. It is based on the Adaptive Information Processing Model, which describes the brain's natural and spontaneous ability to process and integrate our experiences adaptively. The Adaptive Information Processing Model suggests that this innate system of information processing becomes blocked when experiences overwhelm us. These traumatic situations are stored in our brain, where they remain unintegrated and unresolved. The essential elements associated with the event, such as the original scene, sounds and scents, as well as the emotions and bodily sensations, are activated every time a stimulus evokes that experience, and this results in a series of problems in the present.

EMDR therapy stimulates the activation of the adaptive processing system, with the intention to help the brain process painful and traumatic memories. Throughout the EMDR process, bilateral stimulation is used to promote eye movements, as these seem to enable the integration of information.

The ability to integrate and manage an experience depends on the resources of each person, and in childhood these resources are more limited due to the immaturity of that age. Thus, apart from experiences that we would all consider traumatic, seemingly innocuous experiences from an adult's perspective can have a painful impact on children.

EMDR therapy facilitates the necessary adaptations to the child's evolutionary development to get closer to the traumatic memories. This means that EMDR can be used on children and adolescents with a wide variety of emotional problems or psychological difficulties, promoting their improvement and well-being, as well as facilitating their continued healthy development.

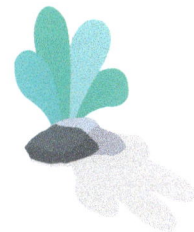

THE EMOTIONAL

It is as if we had a secret garden deep within us, where seeds of different colors, textures and tastes are hidden and blossom into different emotions.

When those seeds germinate, their stems and flowers appear on the surface and express themselves in our whole being: in our lips, eyes, face, in the entire body, inside and out, in the heart and the mind.

The momentum of the protruding stem resembles an electric current that we feel inside us. The intensity or push depends on the emotion. When those seeds bloom, they are very different from one another.

We feel comfortable with emotions such as joy, happiness and love, and they make us feel good. These emotions are contagious and spread rapidly to others.

There is no need for us to talk because with only a look our body's electric current reaches others and those same pleasant emotions grow within them. These emotions have been watered by the pleasant and beautiful events that have happened to us, or by precious things that we remember. They push us to play, to laugh, and to share our well-being.

At other times, seeds that have been watered by terrible storms result in budding emotions that we do not like, or that make us feel bad. These emotions can be fear, anger or sadness. We do not want to feel these emotions; we want them to go away and to disappear. If these emotions have been exposed to a lot of water, they might grow and become very strong. The more we want them to leave, the stronger their stems and roots will grow, and the worse we will feel as a result.

GARDEN

It is possible that our minds find a way to look away from them or to cut the stems so as not to see them. Then, only the roots will grow and, without being able to see them, we may feel confused or may even feel nothing at all.

Although we may not like these emotions, they have an important role because they remove us from people or things that make us suffer or feel bad. We can even say that, in a way, they protect us. Nevertheless, life occasionally makes us live through unintentional or unprovoked situations that are painful or difficult, and we are unable to change them. The emotions related to situations of distress also take root, and both our inner gardens and our skin are drenched in their perfume. The scent of these undesired emotions can also be passed on to others, leading them to feel the same burdensome emotions.

When seized by these emotions, we tend to withdraw: we do not feel like playing, having fun or sharing with others. These emotions emerge when they are provoked by ugly or painful experiences, or by the memory of such situations.

A child's emotional garden must be cared for and tended to by sensitive and experienced gardeners. The best gardeners are parents and caregivers. With their experience and observational skills, they will be able to recognize and name different emotions. They will be able to find the feelings that create these emotions within the body and identify which experiences or memories created them. It is crucial that the gardeners who attend to the emotions are sensitive gardeners, who can perceive which seeds are sprouting, even without the use of words. This way, we will always be able to speak about what has happened to us, both the good and the bad. Proper gardeners water the flowers and ensure that the best situations and happiest emotions flourish. At the same time, they take care not to encourage or fertilize situations that feed painful feelings. A careful gardener will take action with emotions that create distress. They provide love, presence and comfort, and by doing so, the intensity of the pain will decrease.

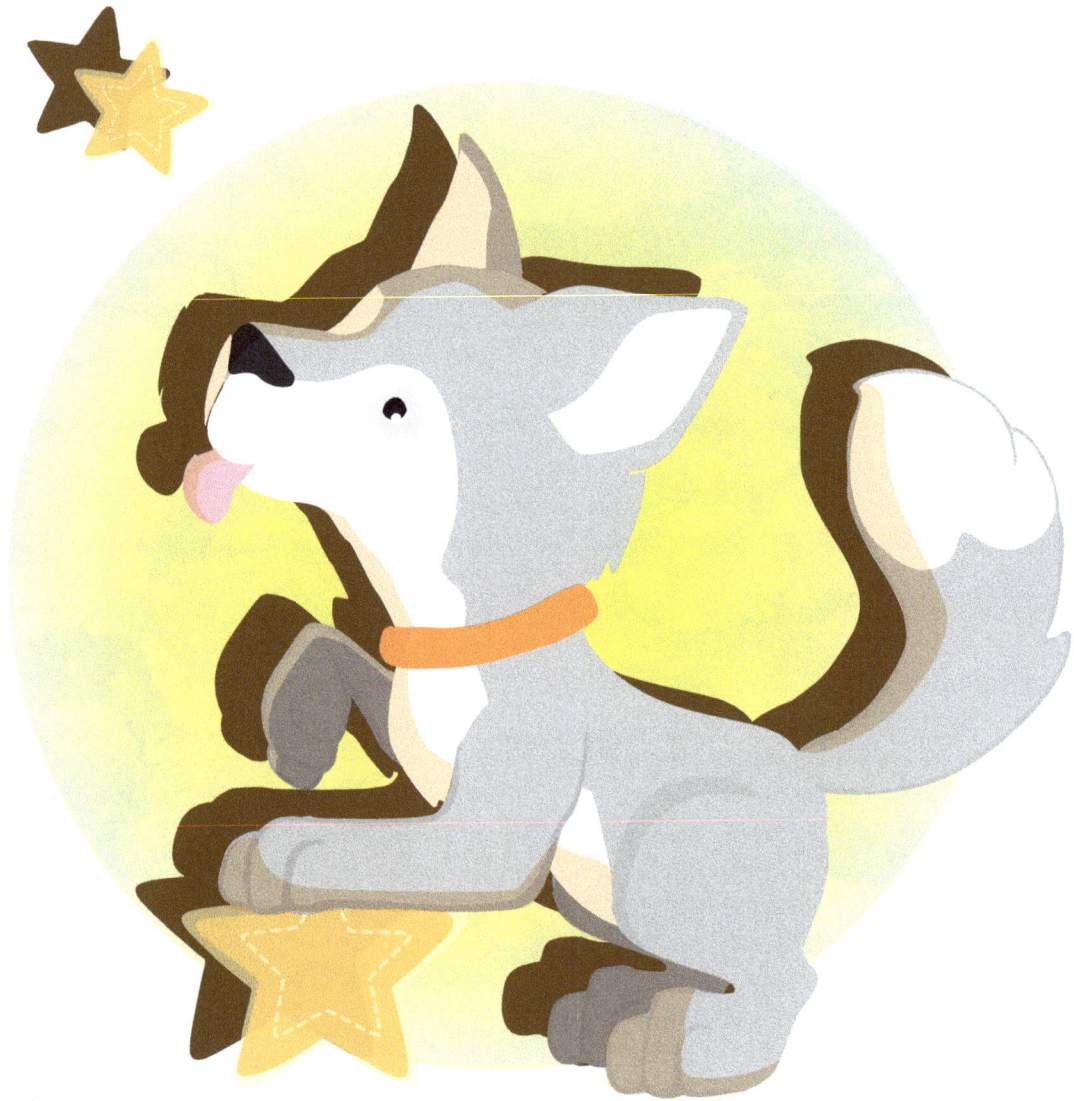

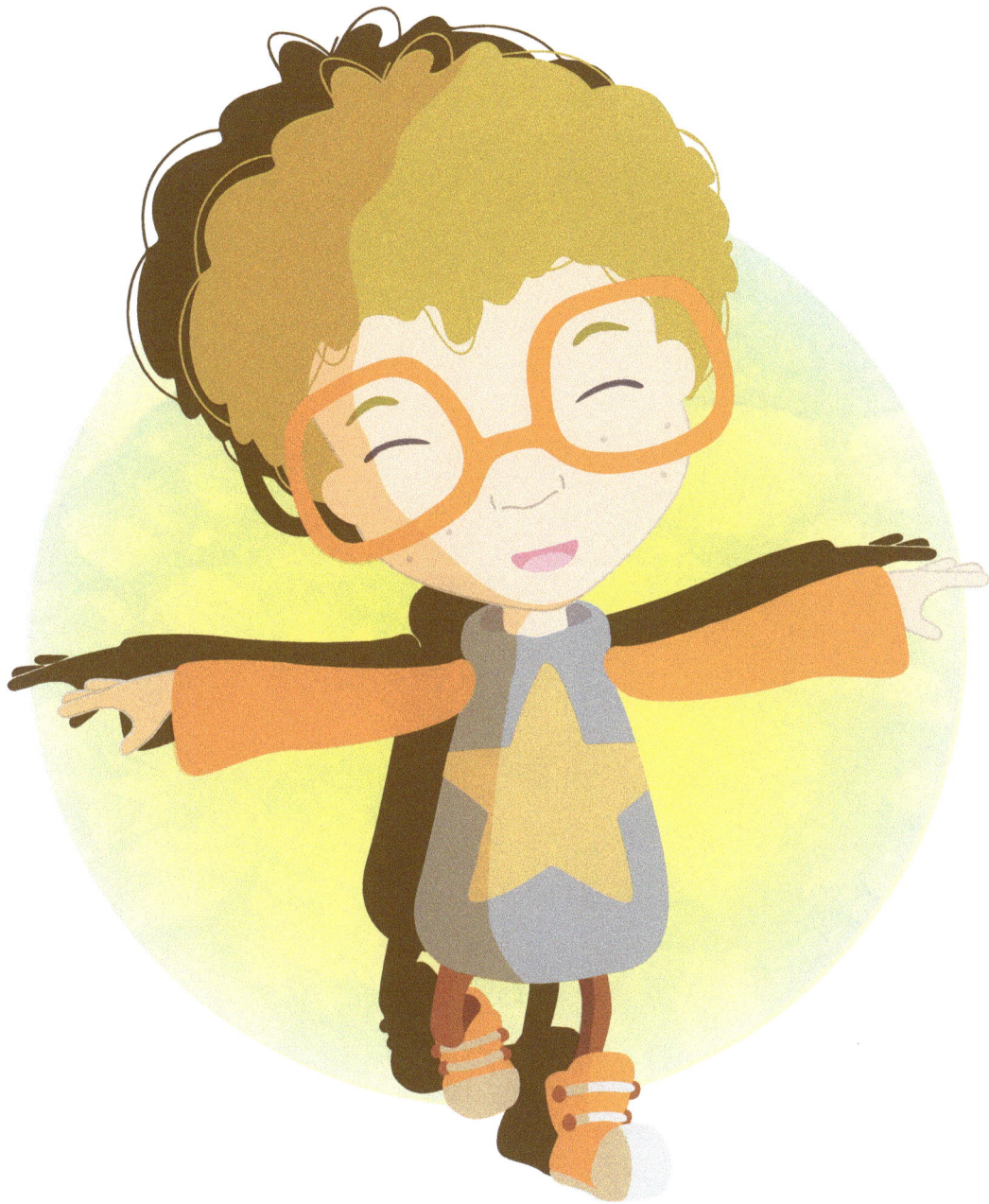

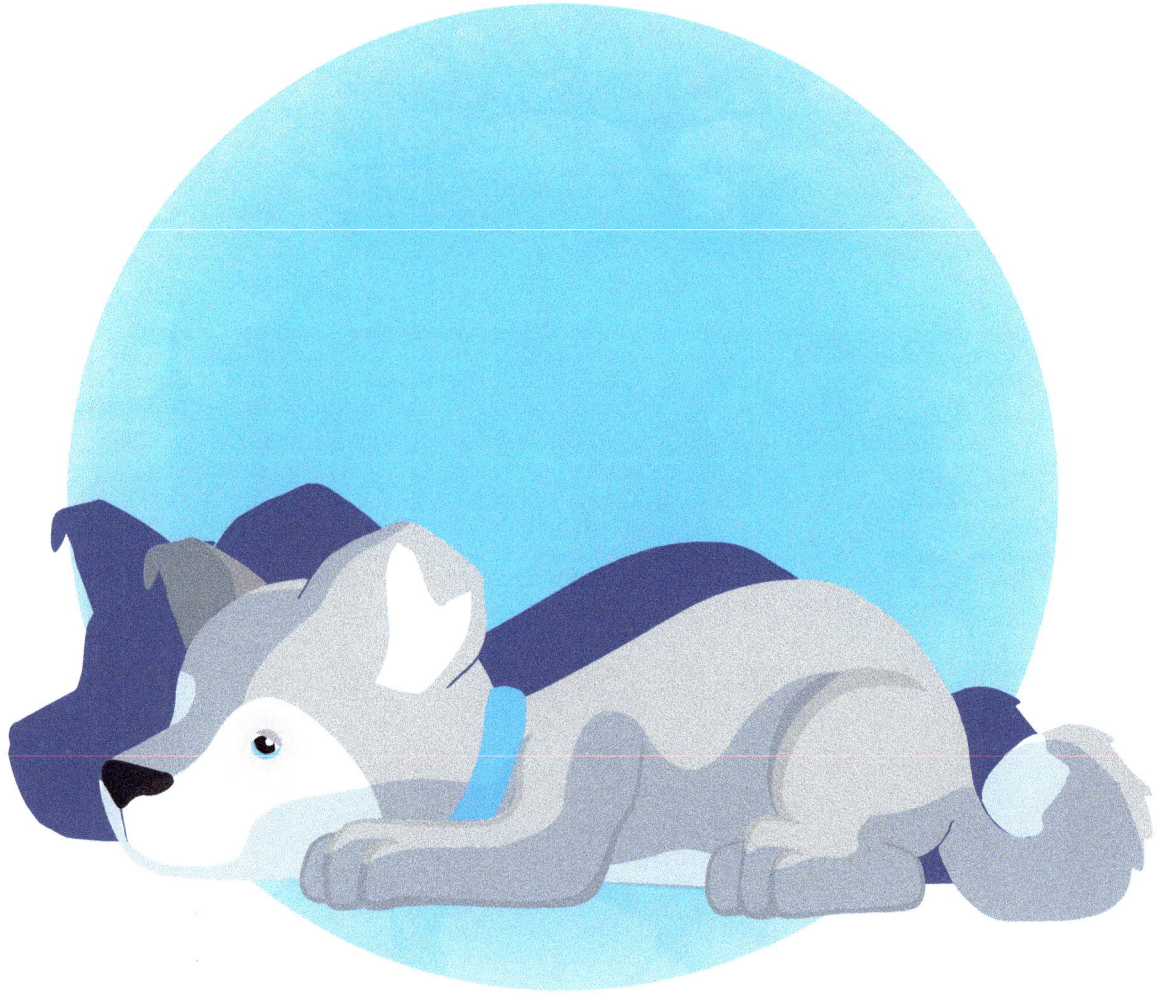

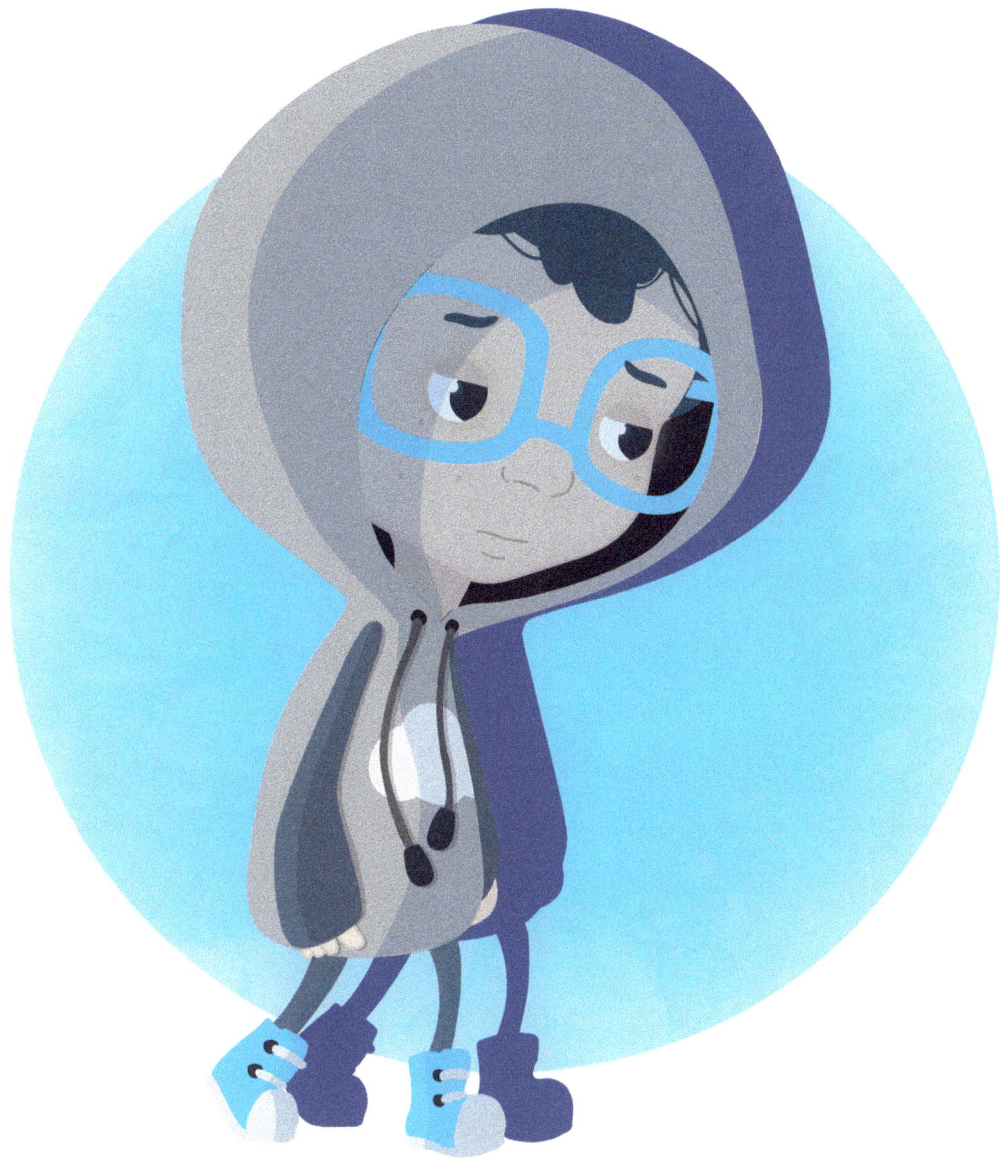

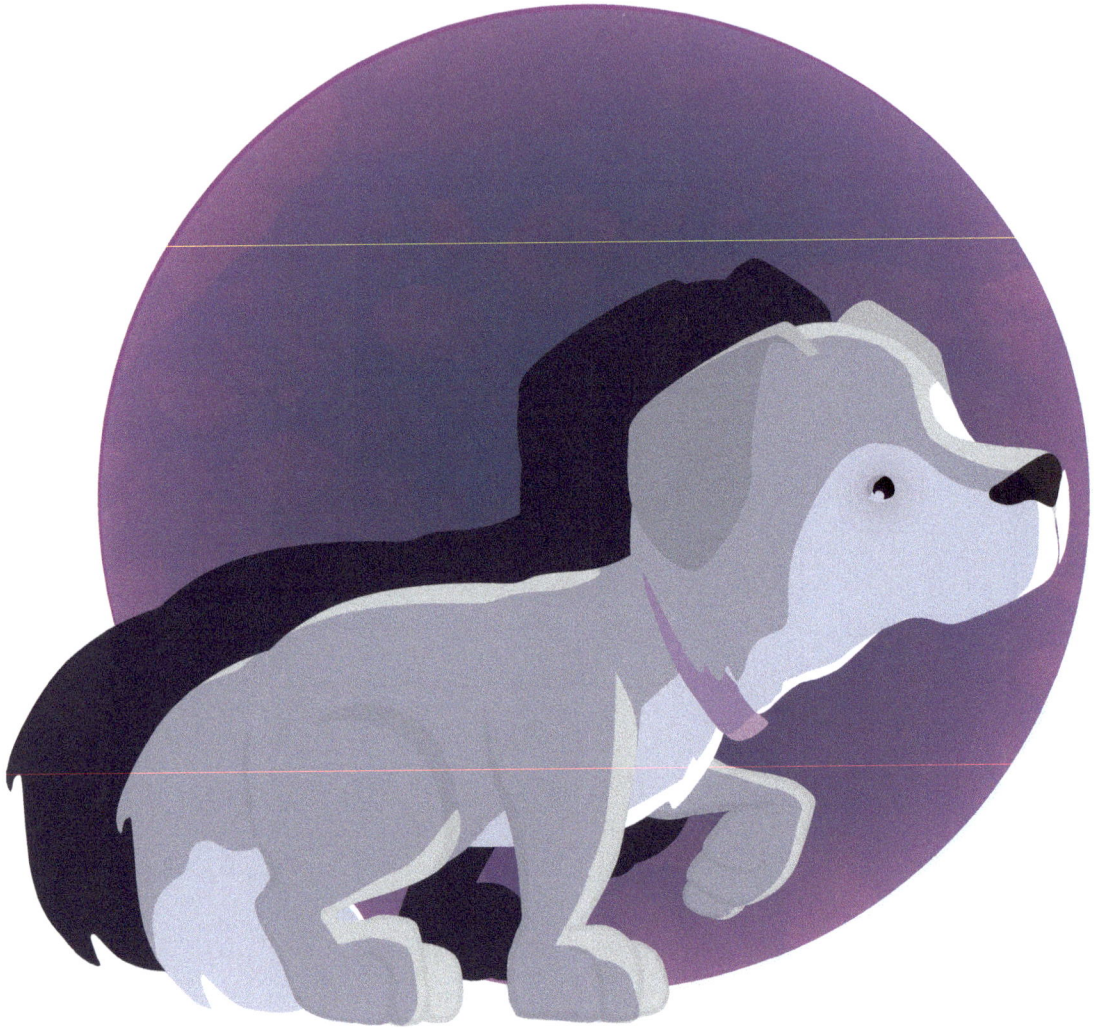

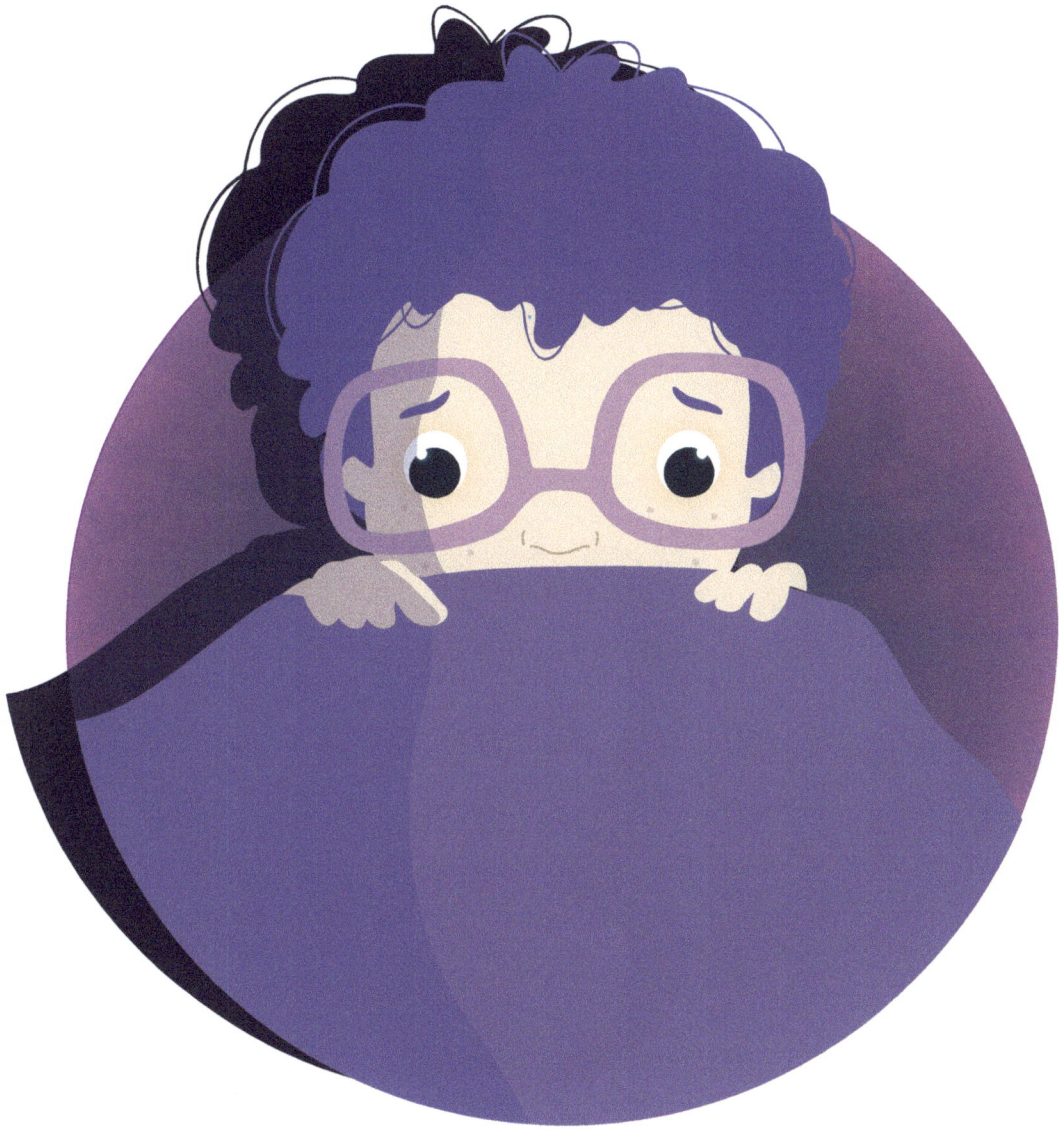

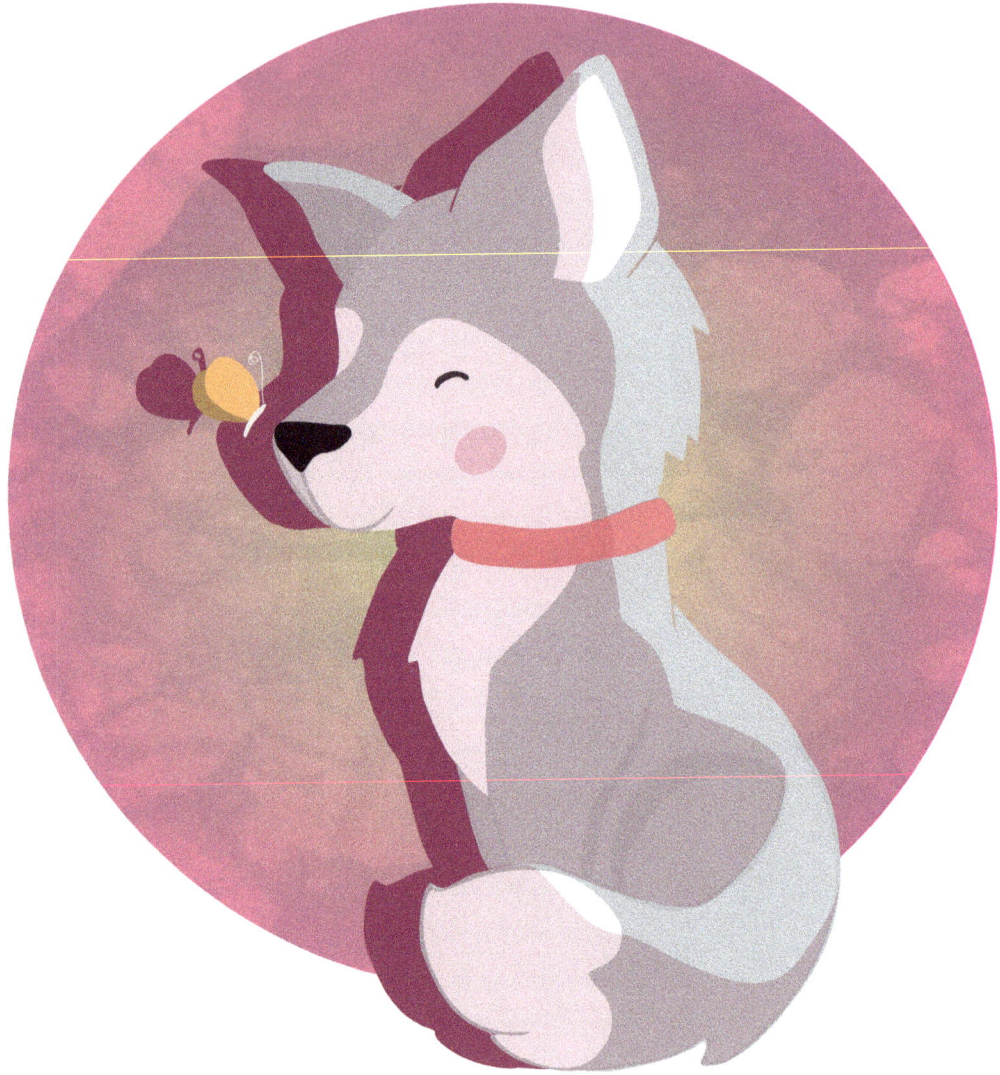

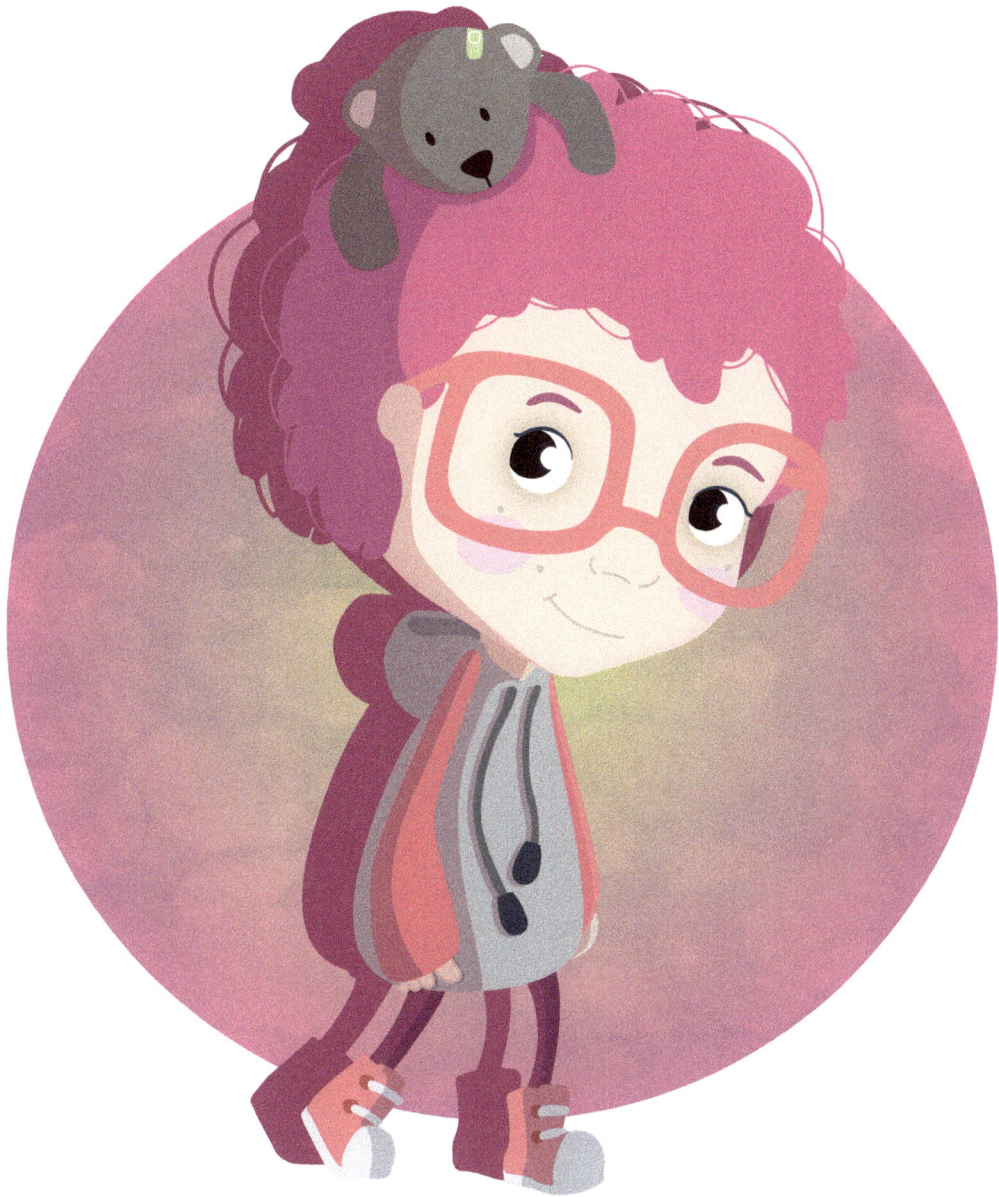

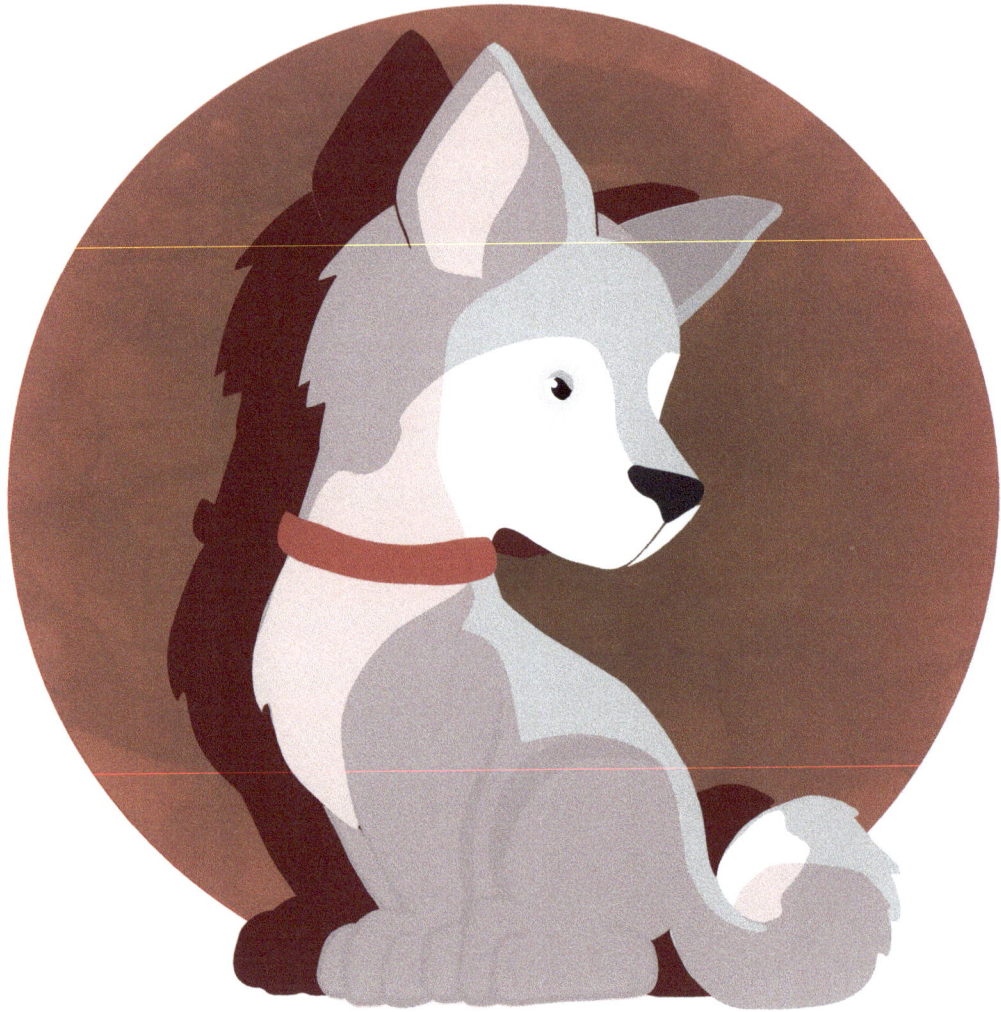

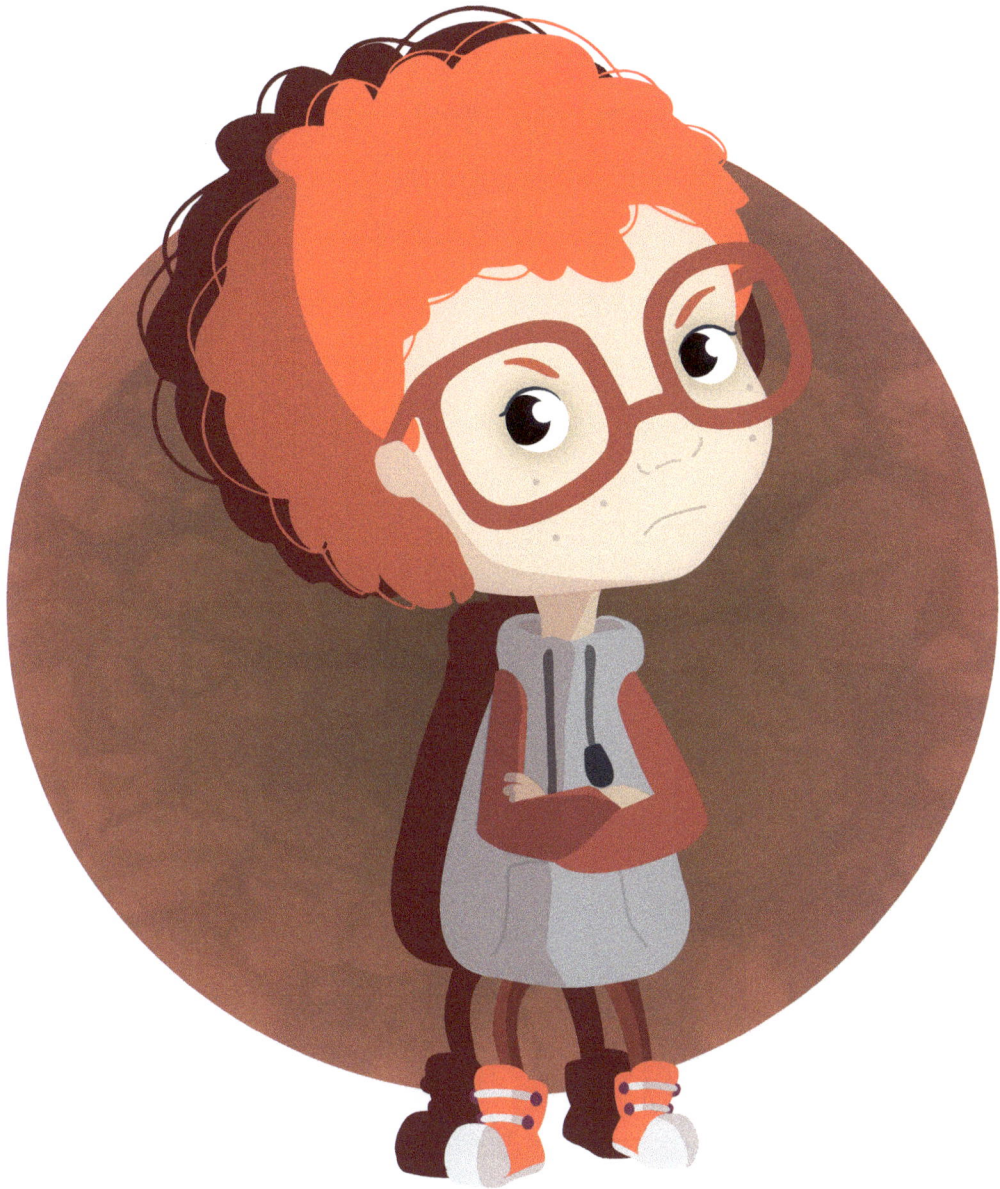

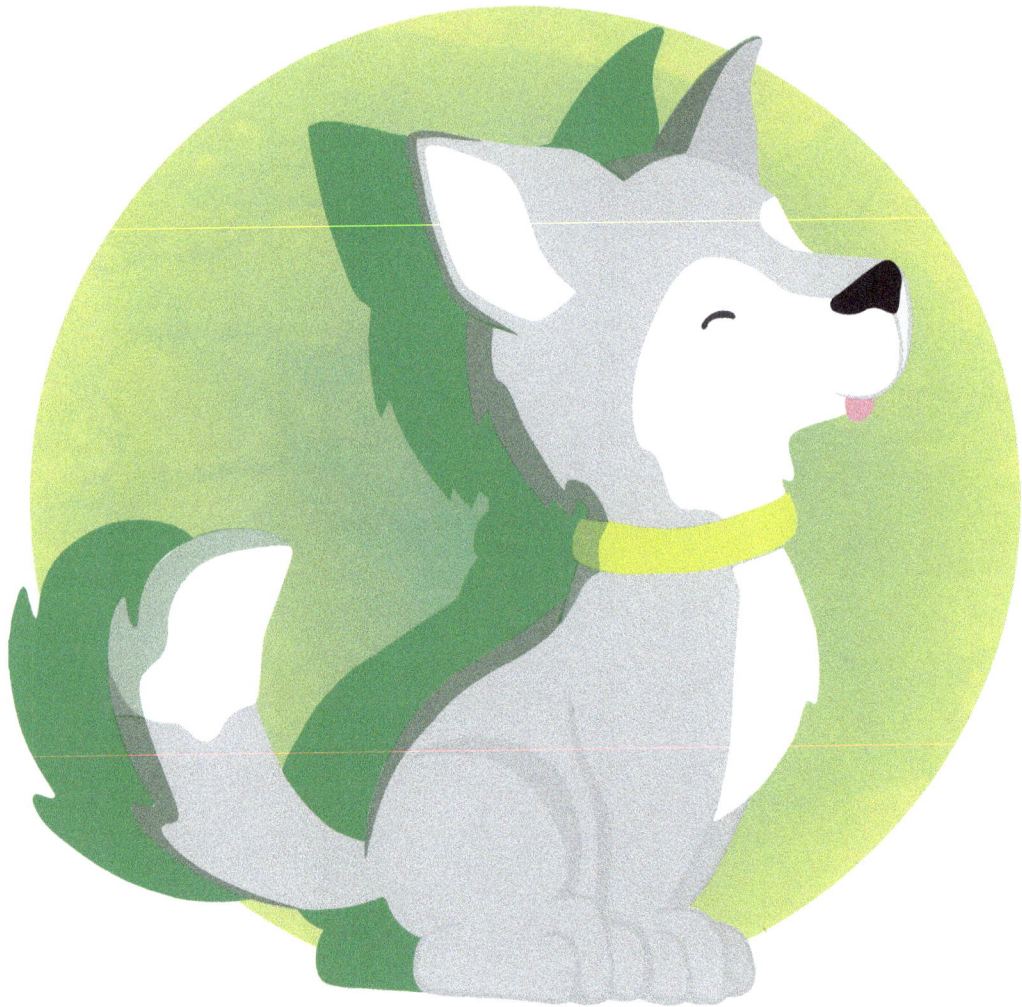

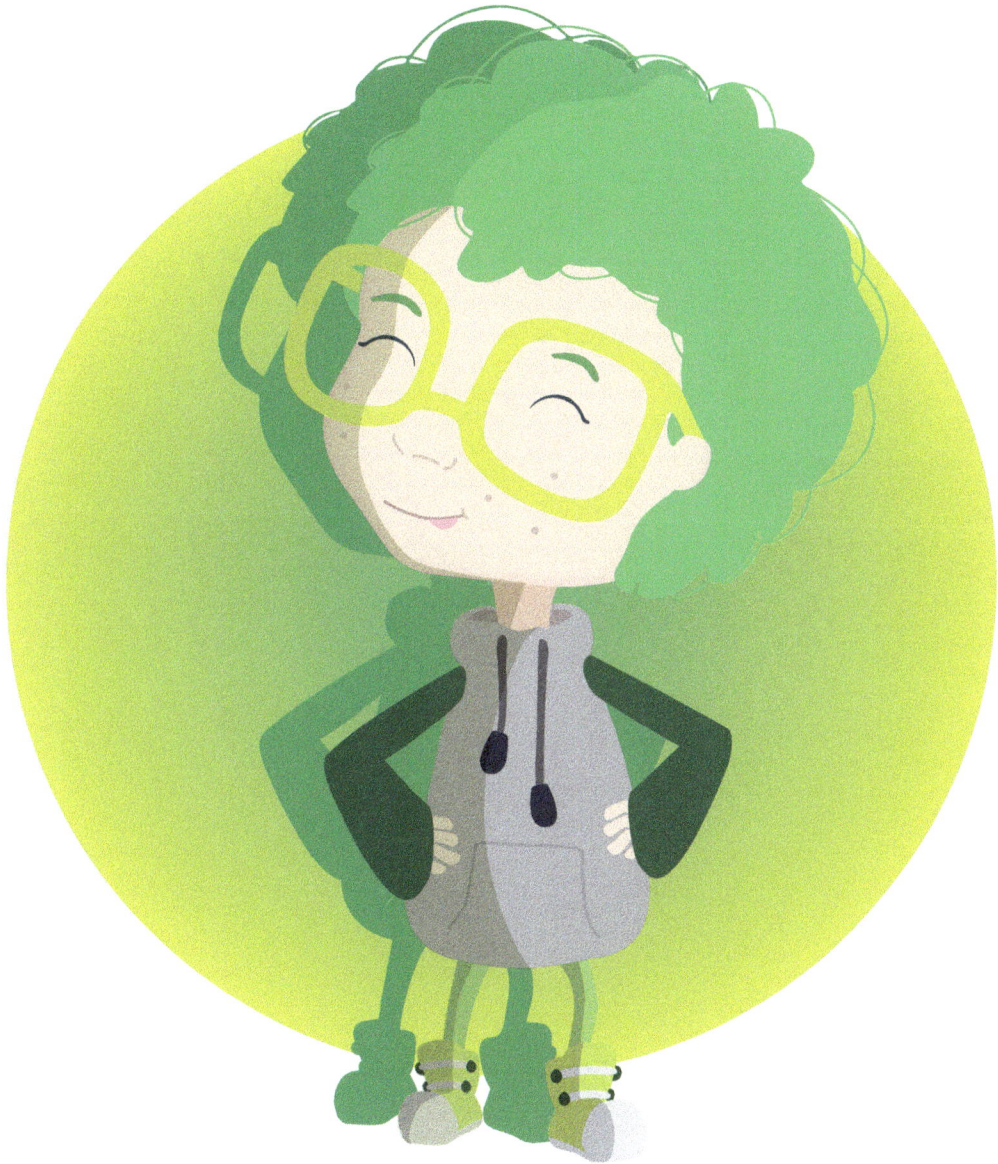

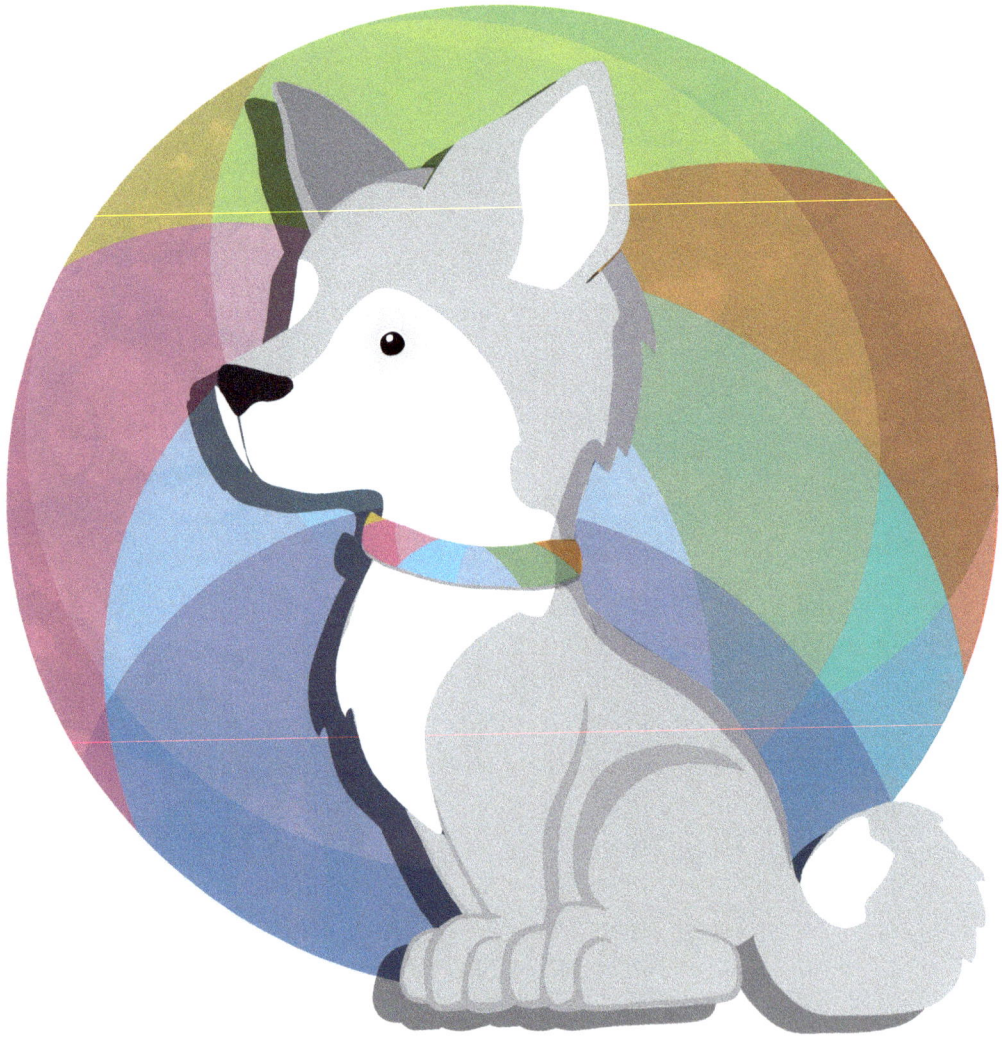

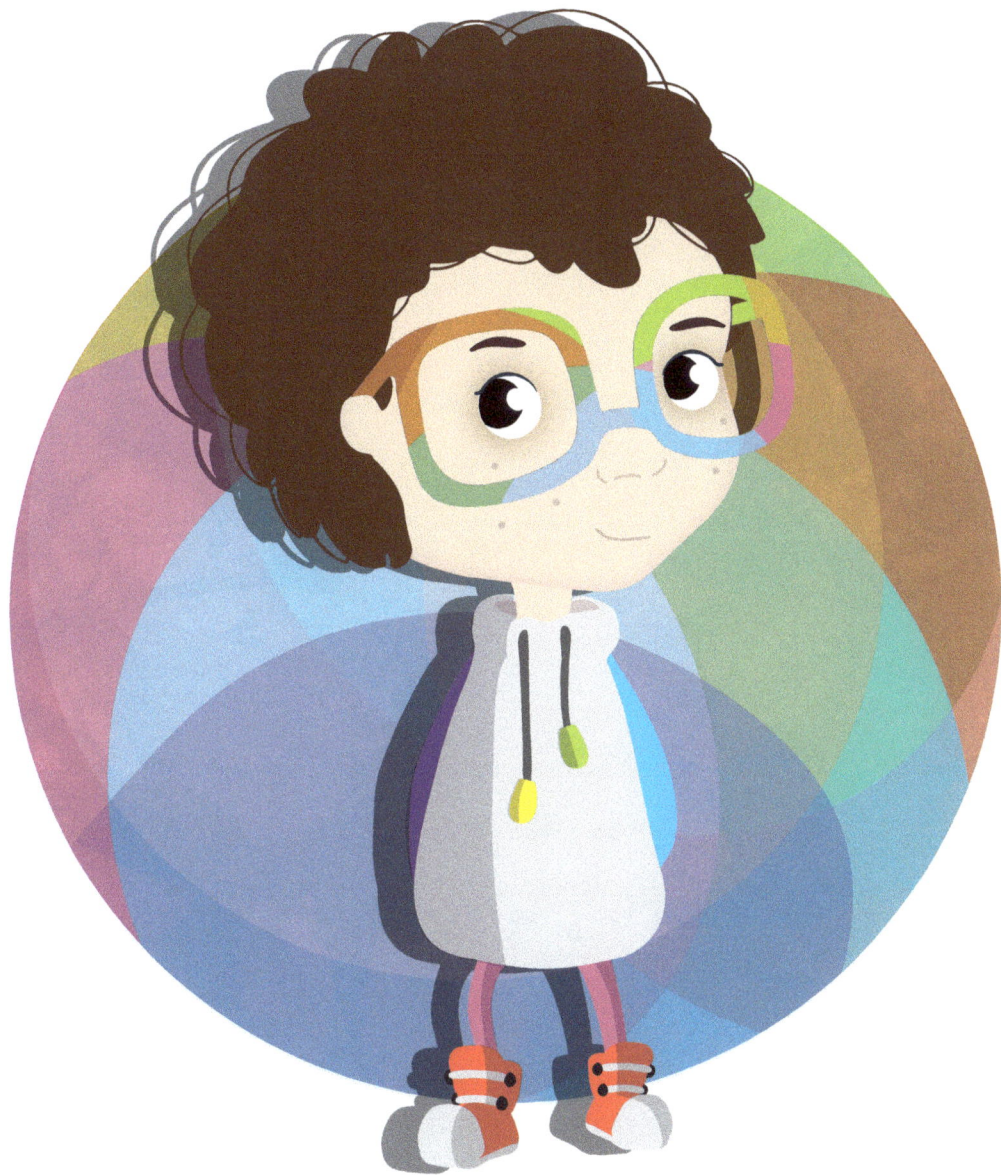

iLLUSTRATiONS

YELLOW
JOY

BLUE
SADNESS

PURPLE
FEAR

PiNK
LOVE

RED
ANGER

GREEN
HAPPINESS

RAiNBOW
INTEGRATION

HOW TO EXPLORE THE EMOTIONAL GARDEN

I present the basic emotions of joy, happiness, love, fear, sadness and anger through the main characters in my children's book.

The illustrations have been designed to facilitate various activities, in such a way that they allow us to explore the child's emotional garden. They can facilitate an initial contact with emotions if we are unsure of where to start.

Among other activities or exercises, the illustrations may be used in the following manner:

HOW to Use the DOG illUStRaTiONS:

The emotions reflected in the illustrations of the dog can be used to bring us closer to the emotional world of the youngest children or to children with difficulty recognizing emotions. When projecting emotions through an animal, we enable a detachment which can come as a relief for children who have suffered an early trauma.

It is advisable to start by going over each of the positive emotions. When the child feels comfortable with these, we then move on to the negative emotions.

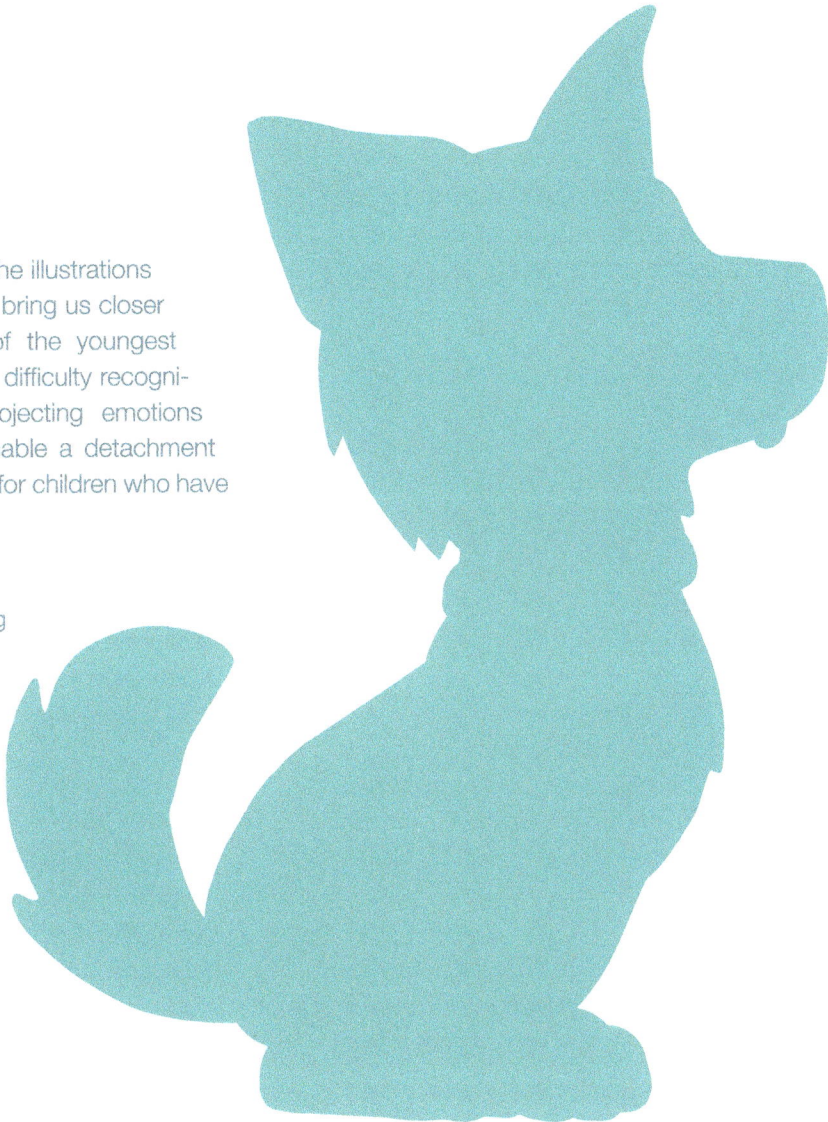

1. We show the illustration to the child and ask them to tell us which emotion they believe the dog is feeling, thus inviting the child to feel the same way.

▶ If they are unable to identify the emotion, we help them.

2. If they can identify the emotion, we then ask them what they believe happened that resulted in the dog feeling this way. The child's response will be influenced by their own experiences, which will be projected.

▶ If they are unable to do so, we invite them to follow our modelling. We are the ones who describe an action that generates this emotion.

3. When the child describes the action that created this emotion, we then ask: "When this occurs, and the dog feels that emotion, what sensations might the dog have within its body and where does it feel those sensations? We want them to locate the positive emotion in the body; we focus on the body and register the emotion. We then ask the child to imitate the emotion in order to establish a physical connection with the emotions and feelings.

▶ If they are unable to locate the feelings, we tell them where we think the dog is feeling that emotion. We can offer various examples, such as joy spreading from the mouth and reaching the eyes, the relaxation of the chest when feeling happiness, and the feeling of bliss in the heart with love.

4. Afterwards, we can ask them if they have ever had an experience during which they felt any of these emotions.

▶ If they share an experience with us, we ask them to recall this positive memory and to tell us where they are now feeling the bodily sensation that comes with that emotion. Again, they can imitate the emotion in order to register it in their body.

▶ If they are able to do so, we ask if they can evoke the memory and if they can now allow themselves to feel that positive emotion and sensation. We invite them to become aware of how they create this state when they bring nice and pleasant events to mind. They see that they are able to create enjoyable states.

▶ From the ages of 7 and 8, we can ask them to tell us which positive thoughts are associated with these memories and feelings as their stage of maturational development makes this possible.

▶ If you are an EMDR psychotherapist, and adequately trained in this therapy, these activities can be carried out in the second phase of the EMDR protocols, which relate to stabilization and regulation. You can, therefore, conduct a short bilateral stimulation set to install this pleasant bodily sensation in the body.

▶ If the child cannot describe a situation in which they have experienced the emotion, we ourselves describe an event in which we have felt that emotion.

5. Once we have been able to perform the most complex activities with positive emotions, we must carry out the same exercises with negative emotions.

▶ Equally, from the approximate ages of 7 to 8, keeping in mind the stage of maturational development and if they are able to connect with their thoughts and beliefs, we can ask them about the ugly and dark thoughts that emerge when remembering an event.

▶ With such discomforting emotions, once the child has located the bodily sensation when evoking the memory that generated the emotion, we should not prolong contact with the sensation in the child's body, as we do not want to drag them into that state. We finish by connecting with the present. We are playing at exploring their emotional garden, something that is not happening to them now but that happened a year or a month ago. We guide them to connect with the present moment.

▶ If you are an EMDR psychotherapist, you must keep in mind that we do not conduct bilateral stimulation sets with negative emotions, given that we could deepen the discomfort this way. We can locate the bodily sensations, but we do not conduct bilateral stimulation. If the child is able to project their negative experiences onto the dog, or if they share disturbing situations that they have experienced, we make a note of them. These can be possible events or memories that we will have to process in the third phase of the protocol.

▶ If you are an EMDR psychotherapist, the previous work of psychoeducation and emotional exploration will facilitate subsequent phases. Without the identification and contact of the emotions and bodily sensations, processing the traumatic situations is very difficult. This is because all trauma, and indeed every experience, is recorded and stored in the body.

6. Once the child is able to describe their own experiences, it is no longer necessary that they narrate the experiences that the dog might have had. We can ask them directly when they felt this emotion and personalize the activity.

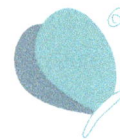

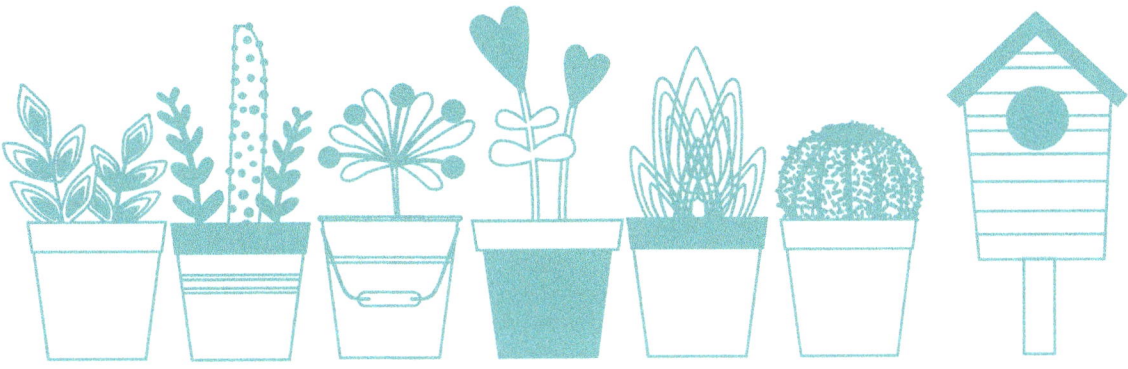

HOW tO USE the iLLUStRatiONS OF the ChilD:

The illustrations of the child can be used with older children, or with children who connect easily with their emotions and can manage the intensity of disturbing emotions.

We conduct the same activities used with the dog. They are described above in points 1 to 6.

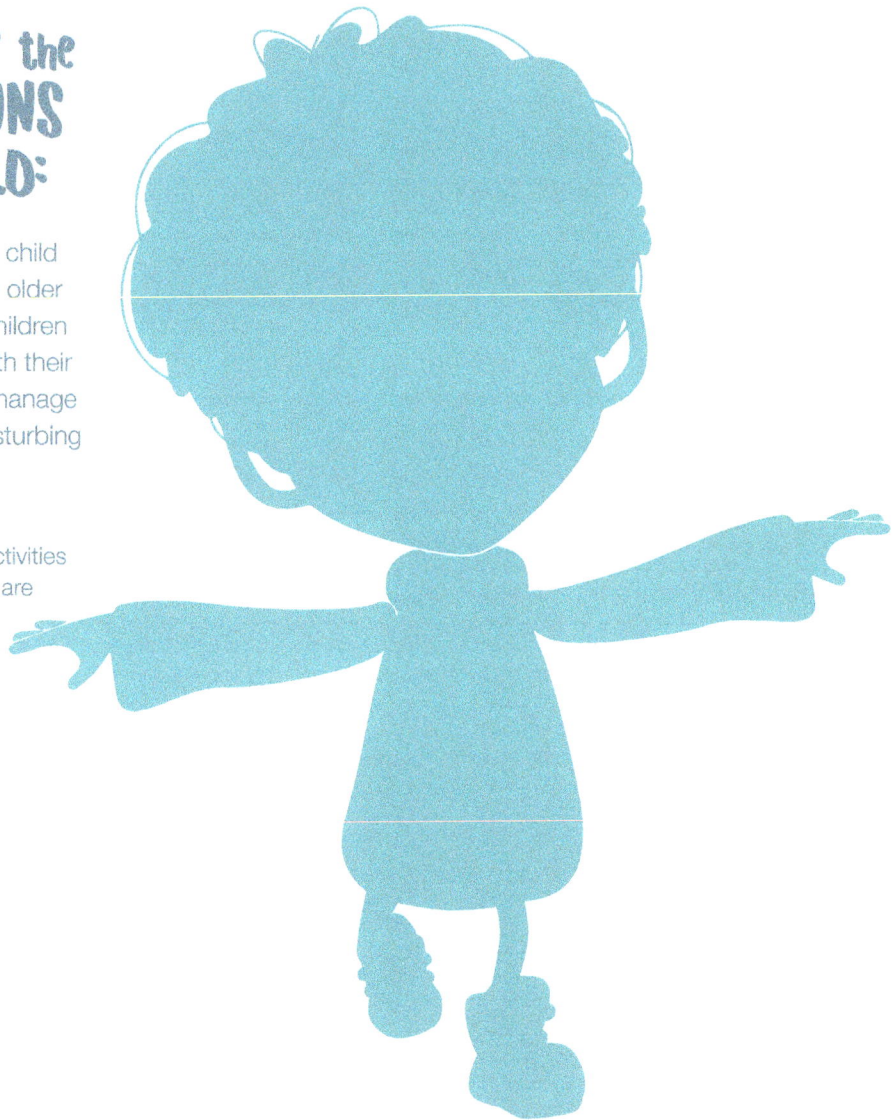

These exercises are a simple way to facilitate contact with the emotional world. A child's mind is concrete and sensory, and by using images they find it easier to connect with their emotions and feelings.

In addition to performing these or other activities that promote contact and connection with emotions and sensations, it is important to incorporate the emotional and sensory content of experiences on a day-to-day basis. We should encourage children to describe emotions, as well as what and how we feel in the body when we experience them. In this way, our children, our students and our patients learn to handle emotions and sensations. They discover that they, like us, also experience the whole range of emotions. All emotions manifest themselves at one time or another, and we do not reject any of them. We do not prevent the manifestation of fear, anger or sadness, and neither do we censor joy, love or happiness. When we allow for the expression of each emotion, we encourage the integration of all our emotional states. We do not reject any aspect of ourselves or of the children with whom we relate. In this way, we facilitate the integrity of the personality that is being developed.

Other uses for the illustrations:

Another possible use of the emotion images is to ask the child to choose the image that best represents the emotion they are feeling or the one that is presently being addressed. We choose the mammalian emotions of the dog or the child, depending on which one we think will be easier for them to use.

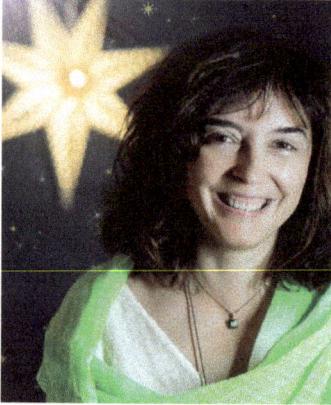

CRISTINA CORTÉS

Cristina Cortés Viniegra is a child psychologist who specializes in trauma and development. She teaches families as well as professionals. It is worth noting that she is the director of the Vitaliza Psychology Center and teaches EMDR C&A therapy.

She considers herself a storyteller. Throughout her childhood, she was surrounded and delighted by tellers of tales. The stories are part of her therapeutic intervention, being a means to display emotions, questions and desires, as well as helping to construct the narratives that integrate the experiences. She is the author of the book Look at Me, feel me. Strategies for the repair of attachment in children through EMDR.

ZUZENE SEMINARIO

Zuzene Seminario Martínez is a children's art educator. She directs, together with Daiana Etxeberría, the Kaligramak Creative Space, where she invests all her knowledge and commitment to favor the development of creativity, imagination and above all, the enjoyment of children in this process. She has a degree in Fine Arts and is a Sociocultural Animator and explorer of the possibilities of art as a tool of intervention and social transformation.

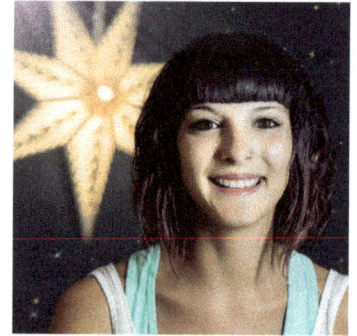

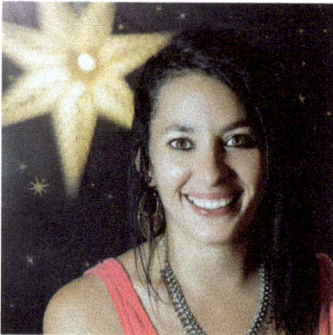

DAIANA ETXEBERRIA

Daiana Etxeberria Santa Cruz is passionate about painting and printing techniques. She has a degree in Fine Arts and a Higher Degree in Graphic Techniques. Together with Zezene Seminario she directs the Kaligramak Creative Space where she shares her way of understanding artistic expression with children. She speaks with them and together, in the language of color, they build conversations in which all expressions are possible.

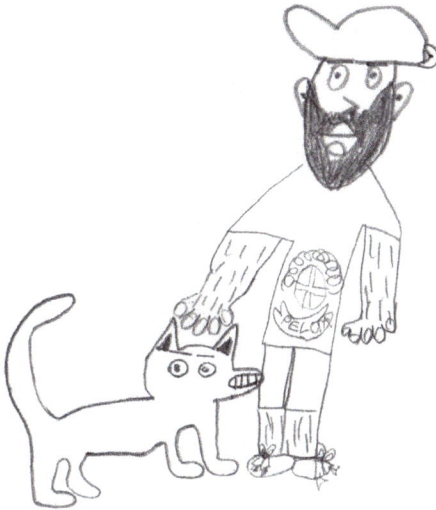

Sketches made by Oskia at age 7,
which served as inspiration for the illustrators.

For the inspiration of this story, I would like to thank all the children that allowed me to share their processes with them and to witness how they had the courage to face their discomfort and to see how their bodies, brains and hearts found a way to recover and continued with their lives in a healthy way.

I especially want to dedicate this book to Oskia and Lola, two incredible, sensitive and courageous girls who are able to rally all their resources and overcome bad times.

My gratitude to Joanne Morris and Michel Silvestre, my EMDR C&A.mentors, for having believed in the manuscript from the start.

My heartfelt thanks to Dainana y Zuzene for finding and creating the illustrations I was looking for before I could even imagine them.

ISBN: 978-1-912764-25-9

Printed by Lightning Source POD

Published by: Academic Conferences and Publishing International Limited, Reading, RG4 9SJ, United Kingdom, info@academic-conferences.org

Available from
www.academic-bookshop.com

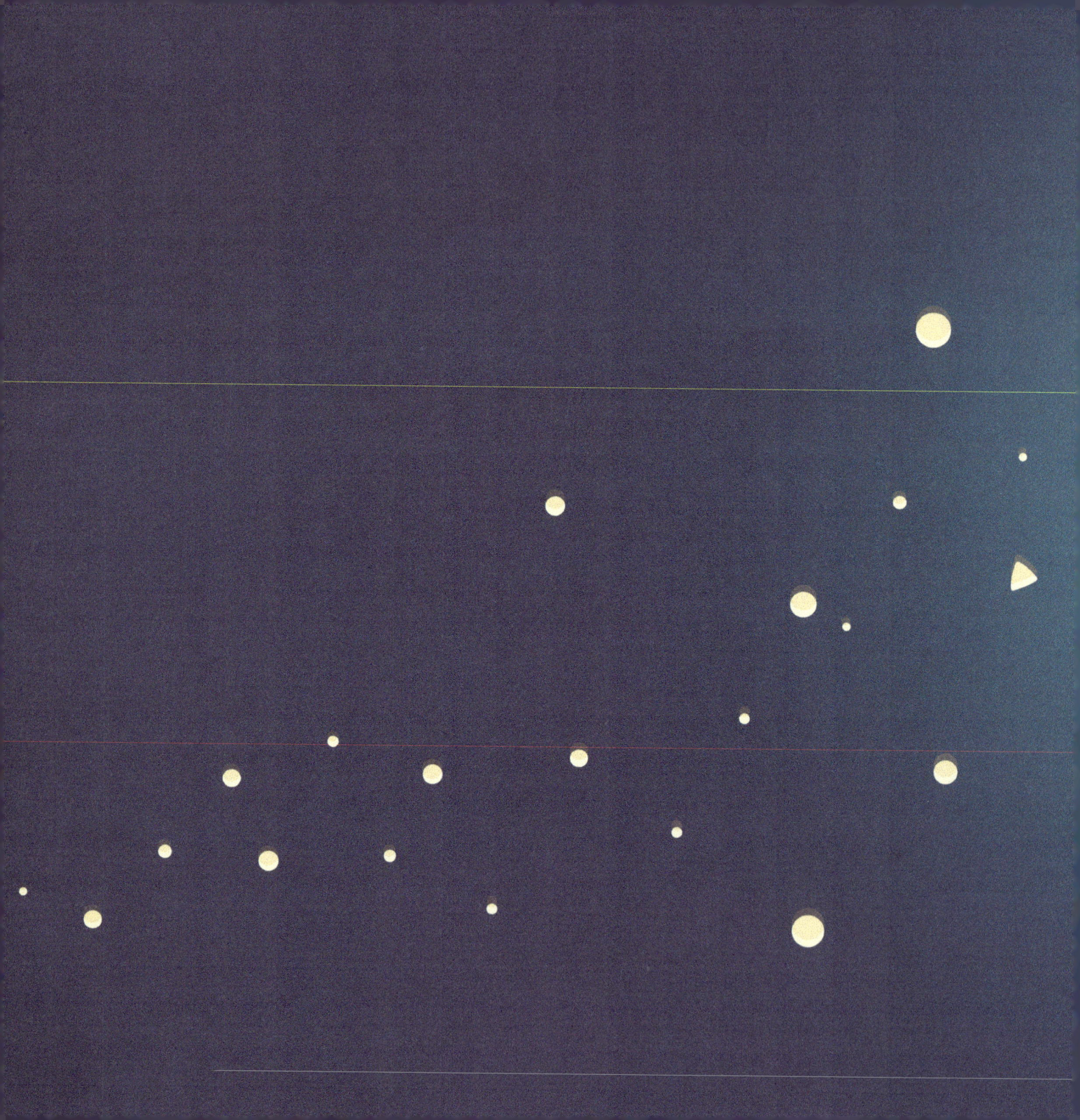

www.ingramcontent.com/pod-product-compliance
Lightning Source LLC
Chambersburg PA
CBHW051257110426
42743CB00053B/3497